THE GIFT OF SECOND CHANCES

WHEN SHAME ISN'T ENOUGH:
SEEKING FREEDOM FROM ADDICTION

THE GIFT OF SECOND CHANCES

When Shame Isn't Enough:
Seeking Freedom From Addiction

—

patricia steele

MISSION POINT PRESS

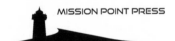

MISSION POINT PRESS

Published by Mission Point Press
2554 Chandler Rd.
Traverse City, MI 49686
(231) 421-9513
www.MissionPointPress.com

ISBN: 978-1-950659-09-8
Library of Congress Control Number available upon request.

Printed in the United States of America.

DEDICATION

———

To all those who have been harmed by my behaviors
I am truly sorry. To the people in my life who have
remained steadfast in support of my recovery, I thank
you from the bottom of my heart.

FOREWORD

———

"Even when we do wrong, accountability is helpful, compassion is helpful, apology and forgiveness are helpful, but shame is not."

–Psychologist and author Debra Campbell

I recall reading an article by Debra Campbell around the time I met Patty Steele. The passage struck me because Patty made a strong impression when she first walked into our non-profit addiction treatment center hoping to work with addicts. Before our meeting, all I knew about Patty was she spent several years in prison. After her release she worked with a program coaching older Americans on vocational skills. Those scant details did not prepare me for my encounter with Patty, who appeared a vibrant, passionate and self-assured individual.

The dissidence between my expectations and the reality was curious to me. I reflected on why my assumptions presupposed a version of Patty that was meek, broken and in need of rehabilitation. Eventually, I concluded that my own bias, my own prejudice had infiltrated what I would typically consider a non-judgmental disposition. How could that be? I work with addicts every day. Eventually

I realized that my assumptions seemed to develop around the concept of shame.

Even if Patty was as "put together" as she appeared to me that day, I fully expected to be witness to her shame. That would support my narrative. Where was the low-hanging head and lack of eye contact I found so familiar in others I counseled? Where was the apologetic tone as she discussed her history? Where was the amplified expression of gratitude when we offered her the unpaid position? I was struck by the lack of shame present that day, at least the outward expression of shame.

As the CEO of Addiction Treatment Services in Traverse City, Michigan, I have seen thousands of people struggling from addiction. The office is located a half hour from Patty's home. Most of these individuals carry the common thread of a blanket of shame. Even my own past drug use, despite never being treated or in the legal system, is challenging to discuss. That is because of judgments I perceive, regardless if they exist or not. That is the thing about shame; it corrodes one's ability to function in a cognitively productive way.

A common adage in the field of behavioral health is that "it's not the addiction that kills, it's the shame." We often wait until the worst imaginable situations take over our lives before we seek or are forced into getting help. The notion of hitting rock bottom is a myth that prevails in our cultural understanding of addiction. We have yet to identify addiction as a public health crisis despite ten percent of the national population meeting criteria for a substance use disorder diagnosis. An estimated twenty-three million Americans identify as being in recovery, yet we mostly relegate them to church basements and certainly do not adequately celebrate their recovery the way we seem to celebrate other major diseases. How often, for instance, do you see a large march aimed at raising awareness or funds to find the cure for addiction? Why is that? I contend it is shame and her sister, stigma.

I came to know Patty over the course of the next four years, and I now understand that shame, of course, is part of her reality. After all, her addiction led her to kill a man - a very good man, she says - in a car accident. In the succeeding pages, you will read about the devastating losses his family suffered, but also the losses Patty had to endure because of her addiction. However, you will also be witness to her strategy to combat that shame by stepping into the discomfort. Shame and stigma only grow if we nourish it. By telling her story, by being a beacon of hope for individuals currently struggling with addiction, and by just living a life of quality and purpose, Patty demonstrates a path to redemption that has little tolerance for the disability shame tends to incubate. It was this assuredness, and perhaps even pride that I noticed on the day I first met Patty. Her shame wasn't immediately recognizable to me because unfortunately it is also extremely elusive.

These are challenging days to work in the field of addiction. According to the Centers for Disease Control and Prevention, the opiate epidemic has led to overdose deaths equal to one aircraft crashing daily, carrying two hundred people. The rate of addiction has remained stable over the last twenty years, yet the consequences of this overdose epidemic since 2012 are devastating. It has exposed the fact that the treatment models we have built around addiction are devastatingly inadequate. It has amplified a deep bias toward "those people" struggling with addiction. Additionally, we have yet to implement a public health strategy that promotes prevention efforts to keep people out of rehab or recovery supports after treatment occurs. No other disease has such a lack of comprehensive strategy, research, or public will to be any better.

If we have any hope of addressing the epidemic of addiction, we must start thinking about addiction differently. We must demand better policy. We must listen to those grappling with addiction. To that end, I applaud the boundless effort that went into writing the book you are currently holding. We need people like Patty Steele to tell their stories. We need to see the struggles through their eyes. We must realize that this issue can touch the lives of a local shop owner, a mother, a friend. In short, lives depend on you changing your perspective. That is the purpose of this book. Thank you for being open-minded. Thank you for challenging your preconceived notions. Thank you for taking this journey with Patty.

Christopher Hindbaugh, CEO
Addiction Treatment Services
Traverse City, Michigan

MY PERSONAL MESSAGE

———

As an alcoholic who repeatedly failed to achieve sobriety, I came to believe I was a failure. I thought of myself as no longer worthy of the love and support of my family, friends, and the community. Optimism was buried under shame and guilt and I'd lost hope. Despair was all that remained.

My story is not the same as all those with addictions. Our paths are different, yet they have similarities. Substance abusers experience feelings of loneliness, desperation, fear, and overwhelming sadness coupled with the belief we are unable to evoke change. We pray for transformation while believing that we as individuals are not strong enough in body or mind to bring it about. Faith becomes fatalism. Mental agony becomes the unvarying state of mind and only our substance brings momentary relief allowing us to feel normal, relieved of dread and stress for a short period of time.

Substance abusers in the throes of their addiction need safe havens where they can rest their minds and bodies. We need supporters who bring honest compassion so that we do not remain hidden in our denial. We need encouragement toward a recovery along with the reassurance that someone truly cares. This support is often difficult to find after frequent disappointments and harmful behaviors. For our loved ones, witnessing our demise is frustrating and wearisome. It is especially difficult without a firm understanding of addiction as a disease. Without knowing how to help an addict, the choice to personally detach becomes appealing.

By the time addiction takes control of a person's life, putting down the substance is the least of the challenges. There is nothing easy about abstaining from a substance that you crave desperately with every cell of your being. However, the harder challenge is learning to live sober amid the wreckage of your life. My own addiction deeply hurt and alienated those I loved. I caused a car accident while driving drunk that killed a man and seriously injured his wife. I served seven years in prison.

Willpower is not enough. If it were, there would be many more successful recoveries. Simply put, addicts need help to recover. New beginnings are founded in safe environments that promote healing and opportunities. Safety involves feeling understood rather than judged.

In my experience, the powerful presence of unconditional love nurtured the strength within me to continue my battle of a lifetime. Without this unwavering connection, I was on the path of surrendering to my disease. Luckily, others had clarity where I had none. They had fortitude and faith where I held only doubts.

Recovery begins with moments of hope. Early recovery is full of discomfort and disbelief. A broken person struggles to pick up the pieces. Shame and guilt restrict us from exposing our inner pain, our affliction. Shame and guilt keep us stuck in the active disease. But where hope exists, new beginnings are possible.

It is said that recovery takes honesty, openness, and willingness on the part of the substance abuser. I believe it also takes faith and commitment to a process that offers no guarantees, no cure. Recovery takes so much more than one person alone can manage and that is why loved ones and the community are essential. We need supporters who understand that the healing process may include moments of failure.

For addiction to be more successfully addressed in our society, we must better understand it as a disease and build systems that support the process of recovery. We must remove the stigma associated with addiction so that people are less afraid to seek help and give help. It is my hope that by offering you my story, you will have some moments of understanding about how this disease affects an individual life. It is my hope that these insights lead you to be better prepared to support someone in your life who struggles with addiction. It is my prayer that some of you will be in a position to educate others and build systems of support for addicts within every community. It is my belief that with compassion and understanding we can help far more addicts find a way to build lives of meaning and joy.

Where there is a village, hope remains.

–Patty Steele

Note to readers:
The names of most inmates and the family in the fatal car wreck have been changed to protect their anonymity.

ACKNOWLEDGEMENTS

———

Writing this book was daunting. It was only accomplished with encouragement and collaboration from some special people.

Anne Stanton, thank you for believing my experience could positively impact the lives of others. Thank you for believing that by putting my pen to paper and sharing my story of active alcoholism and recovery, I might help another addict or their loved one.

My brother, Bob Sornson, an accomplished author and steadfast supporter, your skill and efforts enhanced and polished my work. Thank you for your endless love and thoughtfulness which continue to brighten my world.

And to my editor and friend, Jennifer Carroll, you listened to the details of my tragic journey with addiction without criticism and offered only compassion. You taught me to be forthright and fearless with my writing while urging me to be gentle and forgiving of myself. You gave an aspiring author with little confidence in her abilities the courage to write a book filled with intense emotion and honesty. You have all my gratitude; this book could not have been written without you.

CHAPTER ONE

Rock bottom.

Awakening in pain and shock in a hospital bed, learning of the accident.

A lawyer arrives; a man has died.

Handcuffs, jail, prison.

Rock bottom. Again.

For addicts, rock bottoms are considered events so horrible, so cataclysmic, so painful that somehow the substance abuse must stop. It must. It's impossible to live with this level of shame, pain and humiliation. And then we keep on digging, finding the next level of pain and shame.

For me, each new rock bottom was another reason to drown myself in drink. I had to stop feeling and the bottle gave me momentary relief. I could not imagine living with the shame and yet I continued down the path to deeper rock bottoms. It was not a life I wanted. I needed it all to end.

I can't say how or when this disease took over my life. I viewed myself as a typical middle-class mother, wife, daughter, sister and friend. A social drinker. I believed I could choose when and how much I would drink, and I did not recognize the progression of my addiction. I liked drinking, a lot. I never thought I had a problem before it seized control. It was my comfort, my frequent friend, sometimes my only friend.

My middle-class parents were heavy social drinkers; in truth, as I understand in retrospect, alcoholics. I grew up in Detroit. My father was an attorney, my mother stayed at home with seven kids. I was the baby. As my older siblings' lifestyles of social drinking began to mimic that of my parents, I observed and knew I would not make the same mistakes. The seeds of familial addiction were everywhere for me to see. But I never saw the pattern and even if I had, I'd never believed it could affect my life.

As a child, I did not question my parents' consumption of alcohol. All the adult fun in our home included alcohol. I watched my parents entertain with cocktails, highballs, and the clinking of glasses. Happy hour was a ritual at our summer cottage. The neighbors took turns hosting this nightly event. I witnessed their enjoyment, and I heard their laughter. I watched most of my older siblings enjoy the rite of passage to adulthood by joining the ranks of the drinkers.

My own first drink of alcohol was at age eleven, a little girl who wanted to understand what the excitement was all about. I secretly opened the liquor cabinet above the refrigerator. It held the many bottles of liquor, all shapes, sizes and colors. I poured a little of each open bottle into a drinking glass, covered it with Saran Wrap and hid it outside under a bush. The following night, when my parents were not at home, I retrieved the glass. I took it back into the kitchen, unwrapped the plastic and held it under my nose. The smell was revolting. I plugged my nose and gulped it down. For a moment I felt like I was going to vomit, but that soon passed. I began to feel warm and relaxed, even a little light-headed. I liked the sensation.

At eighteen I began drinking regularly. College included weekend binge-drinking that didn't stop until last call. I married an alcoholic at twenty-one. We worked hard and partied hard with friends. I drank regularly throughout my twenties, thirties and forties. My husband drank almost every night, I joined in on the weekends and eventually much more frequently. My only brief moments of abstinence were during my three pregnancies.

It was our normal. Compared to my husband and many family members, I saw myself as one of the lighter drinkers. In our social circles I was no different from our friends. We laughed at the stupid behavior of others and occasionally our own. When someone we knew drank too much, had ugly fights, or was arrested for Driving Under the Influence, it was their problem.

I began to realize my drinking might be a problem in my forties. I wanted stronger drinks and drank more frequently during the week. It wasn't just social drinking anymore. When going out with friends, I would jump-start the evening of drinking with my favorite vodka and orange juice concoction at home. I did this secretly, which became a pattern. Once I started drinking, it was like turning on a switch that could not be turned off until the night ended, and I went drunkenly to bed.

I still don't know when the desire became a habit or when the habit became an active disease. It occurred without my realizing what was happening or that this problem, this disease, was taking over my life. My addiction progressed and shaped a path of destruction and suffering for me, those I loved, and other innocent people I was yet to know.

* * *

The fatal accident was close to my home in northern Michigan, on December 12, 2007. The crash killed Alan Jones of nearby Lake Ann and seriously injured his wife. They were a retired couple with four adult children all living in nearby communities. The accident and its aftermath were a black-out for me. I crossed the center line in my vehicle while driving drunk and hit the Jones' vehicle head-on. My blood alcohol content was four times the legal driving limit.

My leg was severely damaged in the accident and required two operations. My consciousness did not return until two days later in the hospital. I was confused, terrified, not knowing what happened to get me there. My children were at my bedside. They told me of the accident and the death of Mr. Jones. I saw the devastation in their eyes, and I knew there was no way to console them.

After six days I was released from the hospital. Before the accident I had pushed away my second husband and isolated myself from family and friends. No one contacted me. My boys were still in their teens and my daughter, Sara, was just a few years older. They were afraid, sad, and angry. I was also scared and sharp pain radiated through my injured leg, but the drugs helped some. We had Christmas together at home with my bed set up in the living room as a makeshift medical station. I had killed a man, seriously injured his wife, and stolen them from their family. I could now only pray for their forgiveness. All day I feared the knock on the door, wondering when the police would show up. Christmas was solemn, no laughter or stories. The police arrived the next day.

I was arrested on December 26 and charged with Operating While Intoxicated Causing Death, Operating While Intoxicated Causing Serious Injury, DUI Second, and Open Intoxicants. My children and a niece were there to watch as I was handcuffed and placed in the back seat of the squad car.

I spent the next two days in jail. My leg throbbed constantly despite my taking pain medication. The experience was lonely, but I'd been lonely before. However, being in jail was demeaning and degrading to another level. I saw how they looked at me. I felt worthless beyond my words to express. I was released on a $50,000 bond and sent home with conditions of drug and alcohol testing. My leg was a mess, my car destroyed, and I'd been arrested and jailed. My suffering consumed me. My children were ashamed and fearful. My addiction called me to drink, but it was not possible. The court had ordered I take an Ethyl Glucuronide urine test every four days for the detection of alcohol in my system. If I consumed alcohol, I would return to jail. I was allowed to take Norco, a strong opiate, for my leg. It anesthetized my mind along with my body and I welcomed these moments of numbed relief.

For years my relationships had deteriorated with my addiction. I failed to guide my daughter in a thoughtful, parental way. I neglected my boys and they started to find trouble of their own. As painful as it is to admit, my addiction came first. My mind became obsessed with the need to drink. I wanted a drink all times of the day. I had no strong friendships; my previous relationships were destroyed. I felt alone after two broken marriages and a family with its own drama. My twin brother died years before in a drowning accident, another brother had taken his own life. I told myself I had many excuses to drink.

Three years before the fatal accident, I was charged with a first DUI. I blacked out while driving, crashed into a parked car, and left the scene. Someone recognized me from my small community. The police found me at home still drinking. I never realized I hit the other car. I had no memory of driving home in my seriously damaged van.

I felt truly ashamed when the news of my accident became public. With a serious dose of hypocrisy some family members spoke behind my back of how irresponsible I had been. "Drink at home," they advised each other while knowing they escaped the law and consequences many times themselves. I felt demeaned by the process of the courts and public knowledge of my personal difficulties.

I was found guilty of a misdemeanor and I made efforts to address how much I was drinking for the first time. I went to rehabilitation, to Alcoholics Anonymous, and to counseling. Yet I never felt more alone. Counselors wanted me to change, my family was angry about the embarrassment I brought them. The court system made my addiction public, and I was ashamed. But there was no one I trusted enough to share my pain. I pretended to be fine and I believed my counselors to be naïve as I lied to them about feeling confident in early recovery. In AA I sat through the meetings, contributing little or nothing to the conversations. And I always feared that someone in the room could tell I was hiding my ongoing drinking.

I could not open up to anyone still close to me. My pride kept me from sharing how frail I felt. I arrogantly convinced myself I could fix my drinking, but I did not know how. So, I drank alone. Occasionally family or friends came to visit and tried to clean out my alcohol supply. I hid bottles of vodka around the house. Sometimes I promised myself I would not drink until the end of the week, then day, then hour, before I reached for the vodka again.

In reality, I lived a life of denial, deception and secrecy. My family's disapproval weighed heavily on me, so I isolated myself even more. I was utterly afraid, and that fear gave me another reason to drink. My personal pain was intense. Time after time, I thought I'd hit rock bottom, right up to the night when I killed a good man.

CHAPTER TWO

"The alcohol controlled as well as freed me. It initiated most of my pain and then relieved it. It isolated me and kept me company. It was a demon and a friend. It was my path of destruction as well as my mode of survival."

– Patty Steele, Journal Entry, Women's Huron Valley Correctional Facility, 2013.

As my alcoholism progressed there were more rock bottoms. The marriage to my first husband, Brent, ended after I had an affair. My drinking progressed from being a form of recreation to a coping mechanism. It was easy to explain to myself that the stress of a divorce, the pressure of being a single mother, and my own inner turmoil were enough reason to take another drink. I failed to realize the obvious fact I was feeding a worsening addiction. I married my second husband, Steve, soon after the divorce.

Steve enjoyed social drinking; the pretense that I was simply a social drinker lasted for only a short while. As the stress and tension began building, I used drinking to relax.

Steve was taken aback and started speaking to me about how much I was drinking. I was changing for the worse.

My children watched it all. Their mom liked to be in control, but I was drifting quickly into an alcoholic cycle in which I no longer had control. I pushed them away with my words and actions and then tried to pull them back to me with empty promises. Life was hurting for all of us. My disease claimed its power over me. Periods of sobriety became fewer. I began to wonder if the people I loved would be better off without me.

Twice I went into a local thirty-day rehab program. I felt some relief leaving my troubles at home and being with others who understood my challenges. I learned in treatment that my recovery was more than getting past the physical cravings and obsessions. Recovery was so much more than putting down the drink. I had to change the alcoholic behavior patterns that had become my norm. I had to change *me*.

Coming out of rehab, I believed and was expected to return to my life healthy and with changed behaviors. Thirty days away from the world was a welcome respite, but I returned to the same people and the same patterns. On the surface I pretended to be fine, more in control than ever, able to abstain from drinking. But I was never honest about the challenges I was facing. I still yearned for alcohol and the reprieve it brought from my continual struggles. I longed for the cheerful days, fun with the kids, meals, parties. The cheerful days called to me, and those patterns included the relaxation and pleasure of drinking. Inside my turmoil raged.

More frequently I drifted into horrible behaviors. Bad words, bad days, bad weeks. My children watched it all. As my choices grew worse, I protected myself with emotional isolation. I told no one of my overwhelming desire for a drink. I felt trapped in others' expectations of me and I feared letting them down and their disappointment in me. I saw it in their eyes and so I withdrew again. In my isolation I saw myself as a loser and a failure, but I shared this with no one. I craved my drink. I couldn't keep up the facade.

Our household was filled with discord. For good reason, my husband and children were angry with me. I tried to minimize or justify my drinking and they responded with disbelief. Sometimes my children or my husband left the house for hours or days, unable to tolerate who I had become. My husband began spending all his time at the new house we were building; the kids were at the homes of friends. Often, I blamed them for not understanding me, not comprehending the mayhem within me, not knowing how to talk to me, not knowing how to help me.

My parents, friends, and siblings were concerned and decided to pressure me into seeking more extensive treatment. My sister researched a place for me to go. My dad offered to pay for the rehabilitation and the flight, so I went to a ninety-day program in New York. During this rehabilitation I did not speak with my husband at all after saying goodbye at the airport. He was able to call but did not. Three months. The commitment was I would come out fixed, cured, better, dry, responsible, loving, and ready to get on with my life. If you broke your leg and spent three months in the hospital, you could reasonably expect a healthier leg upon your release. But at rehab I felt alone, deserted. Those who I wanted to understand were not part of my treatment. They were far away and not speaking to me. For plenty of good reasons, which I could not shoulder, the people I loved were disgusted with me.

While at the rehabilitation center in New York, I received divorce papers in the mail from my second husband. Another failure and my fault. I told no one of my pending divorce with less than two weeks to go in the process. The last days of rehab were a blur, seeing the world through the shield of my isolation.

I'd become a total incompetent as a mother, wife, and woman. I failed everyone and I couldn't stop drinking. In the six years of our marriage, Steve and my kids endured my three trips to rehabilitation and two stints in a psychiatric ward for attempting to end my life.

I despised myself for the pain I was causing my family and I believed I wasn't worthy of their love. Whether I tried on my own or sought help, I could never stay sober for any period of time. I felt hopeless.

As I boarded the airplane, I was filled with unhappy thoughts of returning home. I felt overwhelmed. As I settled into my seat, I ordered a vodka and orange juice. I had not considered or pre-planned this choice to drink. My disease was still firmly in control.

*   *   *

During these years I did not realize how much drinking was affecting my thoughts, choices, and actions. Drinking fueled a depression within me, which resulted in a reason to drink more if only to numb the feelings. I sank into a personal abyss as my second marriage fell apart and I watched my children suffer. Suicidal thoughts soon turned into actions.

My suicide attempts were real, but also a plea for

help. I truly wanted to die. Although I dreamed of a life filled with joy again, I didn't believe finding that joy was possible. I believed others would be better off without me.

At the time of my suicide attempts, I had no comprehension of the pain I was inflicting on my children. Years later my oldest son, Brent, explained it to me. He said his confusion and resentment was not about my alcoholism, it wasn't the accident, and it wasn't my going to prison. It was about my willingness to end my life and leave my children without a mother.

I never planned the suicide attempts. I would find myself alone and unable to cope with my emotions. Several times I tried to kill myself by carbon monoxide poisoning. I drove into the woods, found a peaceful surrounding, and hooked a short hose up to the exhaust of my van. Or I tried the same procedure inside the garage of our home under construction. It was physically painful to remain in the vehicle as the air became poisoned. Each time I ultimately opened the car door, gulping clean air.

Once I attempted to slit my wrists. Later, the nurse in the psychiatric ward explained to me I cut them in the wrong direction and not cut them deeply enough. Another time I drank antifreeze only to learn it was the wrong kind. Every failure brought more torment.

I tried to take my life during times of sobriety and drunkenness; drinking gave me courage. When I was discovered by Steve, he reacted in anger. His reaction reinforced my belief that I was bringing shame upon us. I wanted to be held, to be comforted, to be understood. I sought a safe haven and a life free from ridicule.

*   *   *

I lived alone after Steve divorced me. He moved out of the home that we shared before my rehab in New York, but now I had to accept that the situation was permanent. My children could no longer handle being around me. They couldn't bring friends home for fear I would be drunk. They worried that when I drove drunk, I would hurt myself or hurt others. They worried I would succeed in my next attempt at killing myself.

My children left home at different times, each to escape my behavior. My oldest son, Brent, moved in with his girlfriend at seventeen years old. My youngest son, Robert, arranged to move in with a friend's family, also at seventeen. My twenty-three-year-old daughter, Sara, was the last to leave. She wanted so much to help me, but she couldn't change my behaviors. She moved in with relatives and I was alone.

The dreams that once filled our home were now destroyed. Mostly, I drank alone. No longer was I a fun drunk. Even alcoholics want someone fun to drink with. When your drinking stems from sadness, you are no longer fun.

I was frequently alone and efficiently filling that loneliness with alcohol. With little to occupy my time, I decided to open a coffee shop near my home. I worked hard at remodeling a property I owned and getting the necessary licenses. It took me a year of preparation. I did much of the physical labor myself though I still had a few friends willing to help. The activity was good for me, but business was slow, and I worked unaccompanied. This allowed me to drink secretly all day long. I drove myself where I needed to go, and I was rarely sober.

There was a time in my life when I judged those who drank and drove with anger and disdain. I thought if anyone intoxicated ever hurt one of my children in a driving accident, he or she should burn in hell. But my isolated soul craved alcohol. I wanted it more than food. Though I was becoming unhealthier by the day, I hid it well enough. Who might look carefully enough to see the shadow of fear in my eyes? The signs were all there, but we live in a world in which only the blind read braille.

*   *   *

It was December 12, 2007. I spent the day at my new coffee shop near my home. I was proud I accomplished opening this business all on my own. I hoped it would bring change into my life.

As usual, I arrived early to open. I ran the shop alone and worked six days a week. Business was slow during the winter off-season. I thought I might have a few customers and make a little money, but after the early autumn, most of my days at the shop were long and boring.

Though I regularly told myself I would not drink during the day or at work, almost every day I crossed the street to the local party store and bought a half pint of vodka. I hid the vodka in the back room and took nips when I felt the need. My disease was progressing, and I experienced tremors if there wasn't enough alcohol in my body to maintain a certain threshold. I couldn't be around people, much less serve coffee with "the shakes," I explained to myself. I don't clearly remember if I drank at the shop that day. My guess is I did.

It was a Wednesday, I planned to close the shop at the end of the day and take the next day off. In my alcoholic mind this meant that I could drink more than usual since I didn't need to wake early. After work, I stopped at a local store and picked up two pints of vodka. I always bought liquor in small bottles; they were easier to hide. I also reasoned I would not buy a fifth with the intention of drinking an entire bottle. I told myself if I had two smaller bottles, I could drink one and quit. In reality I usually drank all I had.

My routine included rotating the stores where I bought my liquor so as not to appear a drunk to the store clerks. I'm sure this fooled no one. I entered stores in all frames of mind and stages of drunkenness to buy more. Many in my small town were aware of my alcoholism and the stories of my poor behavior despite the pretense. I recognized driving far for alcohol wasn't smart. So, I ended up at the same few places buying vodka over and over.

That night I began to drink when I arrived home from work. It wasn't happy hour. I didn't pretend I was merely enjoying a cocktail. I mixed a very strong drink and drank it quickly. I needed the alcohol to release the stress and tension I felt. Alcohol slowed my mind and lessened the turmoil of disappointment and unhappiness. Quickly the first pint was gone.

Sometimes I spent time with a man named Jim. I didn't care for him much, but I was a single woman who at times desired male company and assistance. Jim could fix about anything, he was helpful. While many people I knew had backed away from me, Jim was available. On the night of the accident I decided to visit him at his home. I figured he was cooking dinner and that I was welcome. I loaded up my dog and kitten and drove the five miles to his house.

Jim questioned me about my drinking that night. He

wanted me to stop. I blew him off with a typical dose of anger. He searched my purse when I was not looking. He found my hidden pint of vodka, confronted me and I became defiant and defensive. He was not going to control me. Anger and fear of losing my alcohol flared within me when I was confronted.

It was a cold, gray, winter night in northern Michigan. Snow was falling lightly. I have no memory of driving away from Jim's house, or what happened during the hour before the fatal crash. I had left his house about 7:30 p.m. The police told me later that the accident occurred at 8:30 p.m. and a half-open pint of vodka was found in my van. It was unusual for me to have an open container in my car because I knew that posed an extra problem if I was ever pulled over. I do not remember the accident. The police report stated I was alert and repeatedly asked to go home although it was obvious my leg was badly damaged. The femur bone was protruding, my ankle was twisted, and I was bleeding. An ambulance took me to the hospital.

Later in the hospital, I learned that Jim was worried after I left and decided to personally check on me at home. He saw the accident scene and stopped to check it out. He spoke to officers at the scene and learned that I had been transported to the hospital by ambulance. He told the deputy that I had a drinking problem. My dog and kitten were not hurt, and he was allowed to take them to my home.

The next two days in the hospital were also lost for me. I underwent surgery on my femur and knee the first night and my ankle the next day. But of those days I have no recollections.

My memory returned two days later. Three faces I

loved were looking down at me, their eyes filled with pain. Only gradually did I become aware that I was in a hospital bed, hooked up to machines and unable to move. My children told me a man was dead because of me. They gave me awkward hugs. My daughter and sons were direct and told me everything they knew of the accident and my time at the hospital. They held my hand, sat on my bed, and attempted to be strong for me. I recognized their pain through my own.

Grief and fear took turns with me while I drifted in and out of agonizing sleep for the next few days. I think I was in shock. Every time I awoke one of my children was at my side. I knew they felt tormented, not only for what was happening to me but for what was happening in their own lives. Yet, they remained kind.

I wished it had been me who died instead of Alan Jones. He had a family of four children and many grandchildren. I worried about his wife, badly injured in the same hospital. Fear and grief, pain and shame were my closest companions. For a week in the hospital I was on strong medications, including a morphine drip. Blessed relief. One day my doctor visited and found me watching the news as it broadcast a report about the accident. There was a mug shot photo of me on the screen. The news reporter said I had been drinking and would be charged for the death of Alan Jones.

My doctor turned off the TV and sat down with me. He told me about others he'd treated who caused accidents like mine. He wanted me to focus on healing. This doctor was kind, he didn't hate me. I thought he should, because I hated myself.

CHAPTER THREE

"I feel worthless and full of shame most days. I have brought disgrace upon my family. I have lost my freedom and with it all my self-esteem. I am considered a criminal by society. I feel a depth of pain within me that I don't know if I can survive."

– Patty Steele, Prison Journal Entry, 2009.

Years as an alcoholic diminished my ability for making life decisions. My isolation continued even after the crash killing Mr. Jones. I was the youngest of five surviving children. My interactions with family were fractious and my siblings and parents stayed away. During the months and years leading up to this accident, I insulated myself from their judgement and criticism. Bad days and hurtful words were remembered through the haze of all those bottles of vodka. But now I found it painful to not have their support.

Shortly after the accident my father was diagnosed with an aggressive cancer. In his last weeks, my father helped arrange a lawyer for me. As an attorney himself he knew the importance of good legal representation and wanted it for me. I was heartbroken by the pain and shame my behavior caused him. His daughter killed a man. In his own way, he tried to help me during the ugliest years of my addiction, but he was often abrupt and no model of temperance. Additionally, I had a problematic connection with my mother. Sadly, her pattern of isolation, drinking, and discontent laid a foundation for mine. My sisters had their own families and their own issues. My brother created a separate existence for his wife and kids, mostly away from the family drama. There were no confidants left in my life.

A few weeks later my father died of lung cancer. I knew my shame was a terrible burden to him. I was allowed by the courts to visit him once before he died at his home in Farmington Hills. I was granted permission to again travel four hours south for his funeral. I spoke of my feelings to no one. I believed that there was no one in my life who wanted to listen. I took my pain pills without fail, wanting to be numb.

My sisters, my daughter and I stayed at my father's condo on the night before the funeral. My leg hurt badly despite my walking cast and the walker I used to get around. The healing had just begun. At the time, it seemed my family barely noticed my pain or injury. Perhaps they were avoiding addressing me and my circumstances. Family members decided to not drink in my presence. I was aware some were not happy I was there, and I was sure it was because their drinking was limited. No one commented in the morning when I had to go to the local police station for a breathalyzer before the funeral. I felt incredibly alone. My father's death and my part in bringing sadness to him broke something inside of me.

*   *   *

The lawyer my father hired was a retired district court judge. What I needed was an experienced defense attorney. I had no recollection of the crash. A witness stated that another vehicle hit me from behind before my car crossed the center line. It gave us hope I might not go to prison. With my lawyer's advice I chose to forego a plea and proceeded to trial, hoping that this witness would somehow mitigate my guilt. But this hope was crushed as her memory of the accident lost clarity.

The months between my arrest and trial were spent at home. My youngest son moved back in with me; my daughter was always close and available. My oldest son kept his distance.

I needed to attend meetings with my attorney and preliminary court hearings. My daughter drove me a half hour to Traverse City every four days for my alcohol testing. I had few visitors. Those who came meant a lot to me.

I had distanced myself from the people in my life, including my family. My mother lived only a few miles away, yet she never called or stopped by during this time. I knew my troubles were tormenting her, but she never expressed her feelings to me. My family members tried to intervene over the years but did not understand the full depth of my problem.

Finally, sober from alcohol though not by choice, I struggled to face the truth. I knew now what it felt like to be truly on my own without the daily influence of liquor. My body was battered, my soul cried out for a drink. My father had died, my brother and sisters were disconnected from me, the people I once called "friends" stayed away. It was terrifying.

*   *   *

My trial began in April of 2008 and lasted three days. I sat at a table in the courtroom next to my lawyer. My children and their father, Brent Sr., sat behind me. The prosecutor was at another table to our right. Behind the prosecutor sat Susan Jones and her four adult children. Many of their extended family members were in the courtroom every day. I saw the Jones family in the hallways, but we avoided eye contact and did not speak. I understood that I had done unthinkable harm to them and they wanted what they perceived as justice. I understood, yet I was hoping to avoid prison. I told myself everything would be all right.

On the side of the courtroom where the Jones family sat were also police and a group of lawyers. They listened carefully to the trial and to the testimony of the witnesses. The police were there to support the prosecution. The attorneys attended to gain knowledge of the case for a future civil action.

On the third day of the trial my mother and sister came to court. I had not spoken to them since my father's funeral and had no idea they planned to be there. When I saw them, I wondered why they came. They had not communicated with me. They did not ask if I wanted them there, they had not told me they were present to support me. During the courtroom breaks I felt forced to sit with them and include them in conversation. I felt I was expected to be grateful they decided to appear, but their presence unnerved me. It seemed to me that they were more interested in a first-hand account of the outcome, rather than how my family or I were coping. Old wounds shrouded our relationships and I questioned their motivation.

The testimony was excruciating. I had to listen to the accident as it was described in great detail along with the sordid details of my alcoholism. In contrast, I felt a deep remorse for the family who was sitting in the courtroom with me. The eyewitness I'd once hoped could offer testimony to the role of another car said her memory was spotty.

On the last day of the trial the jury found me guilty. I was placed in handcuffs and taken to jail. All semblance of control over my own life instantly vanished. I was now a criminal, a convict, and a ward of the state. There was no chance to return home to prepare my affairs. I wasn't ready for this. There were no goodbyes.

* * *

I spent a month in jail awaiting the sentencing. It was a fog. I took strong pain relievers regularly for the continuous pain in my ankle, knee, and thigh. I wanted and sometimes demanded my medication from the jail staff. In truth, it numbed me physically and mentally, so I did not feel at all.

Upon arrival at the jail I was strip-searched. I endured this degrading experience repeatedly in the coming years. My clothing and jewelry were taken from me. I stood naked in front of a female corrections officer without possessions or dignity. Soon I was sitting in a cell alone wearing orange cotton pants and a matching shirt. The clothing was designed for one-size-fits-all and my jail clothes hung from my five-foot, two-inch frame. I was not prepared for this transition. I was a middle-aged woman with a bad leg, a confused mind, and a new identity. Grand Traverse County Prisoner was stenciled on my back.

There was nothing to do but stare at the grey cinder block walls and worry. Time stood still. Later I would recognize this time as one of the first circles of hell. There were many more to come.

After a few days, I was moved into a cell with five other women and later to a cell that slept eight. At times the cell was overcrowded with up to twelve women. Some were forced to sleep on thin mats on the hard cement floors. The women were mostly younger than I was and definitely tougher, many having seen the inside of a jail cell before. Largely their offenses related to drugs and alcohol.

I watched several women arrive detoxing. They lay on the floor, writhing in pain, sweating, hot and cold. No one helped. No one addressed their need for medical assistance. For some of the women it took days before they began to eat, move around or talk with other inmates. I felt a strong desire to do something for these women, but there was nothing any of us could do. We were helpless. And so, we watched or tried to look away.

During my month in the county jail, I met women with signs of mental illness. Some displayed extreme anxiety and confusion about their circumstances. A Community Mental Health worker came to check on one woman weekly. This woman appeared calm one moment and in panic mode the next. She was repeatedly removed from the cell physically by the officers when she became aggressive. She was forced into a restraining jacket with her arms behind her back and placed in an observation cell until she was sedate again. The actions of the corrections officers fueled her fear and she fought as hard as she could. After hours or days, a correction officer would return her to our cell. Confinement was her treatment plan. We all had the same treatment plan of wearing orange jail clothes, consuming bad food, being put in isolation, and sometimes restraint. It was the same whether we were drug abusers, people with obvious mental health issues, others with painful past experiences, or lacking models of responsible adult behavior, lacking work skills, lacking social skills, lacking self-respect and self-efficacy. Deep inside, all of us want to be recognized and respected by others, but I was beginning to learn jails are not about that.

I lay on my bunk bed for a month, sleeping as often as I could. I watched TV and occasionally played cards. The food was disgusting. Everything looked like noodles or rice slop without meat. It was tasteless. We drank watered down Kool-Aid. I had no appetite for life much less this gruel that lacked both taste and nutrition.

Once, I left the jail in handcuffs and foot irons to go to an appointment with my orthopedic doctor. I felt humiliated to be out in public as others stared at me. Returning to the confines of the jail felt safer than being identified as a social outcast. I looked forward only to weekly one-hour visits with my sons and daughter. And I waited.

*   *   *

April 16, 2008, was my sentencing day. I was escorted from the jail to the courtroom in full restraints. I entered the small courtroom afraid and unaware of what was to come. Up to this point in my life a sentence was a small group of words that summarized a simple idea or two.

Now a sentence was to influence my life for the next years to come, choose a compulsory path for me that I could not imagine. In the courtroom, many eyes followed me as I took small steps with my walker, hindered further by handcuffs and ankle irons.

The small courtroom was packed with the Jones family and their friends, several police officers, the usual lawyers, and a local television news reporter. My children were there along with my ex-husband and my mother and sister. When I realized I was to be filmed for the evening broadcast, I did my best to keep my face turned away from the camera, hating the idea of my disgrace once again being headline news. "Don't worry about it. You are pretty," my attorney told me. His words seemed absurd to me. There was not a pretty thing about me in this grotesque moment.

Members of the Jones family were given the opportunity to address the court. They spoke of their father and how much he would be missed. They described the loss of a wonderful husband and father and how I warranted the utmost punishment for my crime. He was a beloved family man. I heard their pain.

The judge offered me a chance to speak and I spoke directly to Susan Jones, his wife, saying to her how sorry I was. I told her that I couldn't imagine what it must be like to lose a husband of forty-three years so needlessly. Beyond that, I didn't know what else to say. I expect there were no words that I could have spoken that would have relieved the sense of tragic loss felt by Susan Jones and her family.

My lawyer advised me that for charges like mine I could expect a sentence of three to four years in prison. But my brain could not fully grasp the notion of living as a prisoner. The courtroom suddenly felt sweltering as the judge prepared to deliver my sentence.

As the judge handed down my sentence of seven to fifteen years, I looked at my lawyer and saw his surprise. I held on tightly to my walker as my fate sank in. I was drenched with sweat and my breathing stopped. I nearly fainted. I could feel the camera behind me, and I was determined not to let it capture my face. I did not look back at my family, too afraid to see their reaction or for them to see mine. I was quickly removed from the courtroom and returned to the jail cell. I now felt protected in jail; the world was no longer mine.

Suicide was on my mind nightly during my last week in the Traverse City jail. I learned of another woman who had recently managed to hang herself in the showers. It seemed like a good idea. Every night while others slept, I crept quietly into the bathroom with two large plastic bags I kept hidden under my mattress. One I would use as the lynch and the other to cover my head, but I couldn't go through with it. I was afraid of not being fully successful; I didn't want my children to have a half-dead mother.

On May 24, 2008, I was transported to the state prison. I was forty-eight years old, facing an unknown world. Wearing an orange jump suit, I left the jail with only my walker and a Bible in which I had written down every address and phone number I could gather in case I might forget.

The transport downstate included three men also from the Grand Traverse County Jail. Their destination was Jackson State Prison. No one spoke a word during the four-hour ride. Nothing in my life prepared me for this experience and I fought down the waves of panic. Who was I, who was Patty? I didn't know any more.

We arrived at Jackson to drop off the men. The prison was large, surrounded by layer after layer of tall fencing and concertina wire. It was imposing and overwhelming. This was the first time in my life seeing a prison up close and I watched through the dusty van windows as the men were unloaded and herded in through the large metal gate. The transport officer returned shortly with their orange jumpsuits and chains. For a brief moment, I wondered about them. Silent all the way on the trip, herded like docile animals into the pen, and no longer wearing orange transport uniforms. What identity will they claim or have thrust upon them during their time in this awful place? But I was projecting; my thoughts were not with those men.

My leg was beginning to throb. I hadn't had any pain medication since leaving Traverse City. I said nothing about the pain during our ride. I didn't think anyone would care. The glorious sunshine of that late May afternoon was in stark contrast to my dark and lonely world. There was no joy or sunshine within me.

The transport officer informed me we were going to stop briefly before arriving at Scott Correctional Facility for Women in Plymouth where I would begin my sentence. He pulled into a Michigan State Police Post where I was allowed to use the bathroom. The officer removed my handcuffs and warned me not to run.

I considered myself, with my walker, my pain, my broken leg, and my shackles on hand and foot. Really? Really? Don't try running away? The absurdity struck me, but not as something funny. It was a road sign, one completely absurd remark delivered within a context that I could not understand. I wanted to say something sarcastic to him, but there was no humor, no arrogance and no

27

wit within me. I was just somebody on a bus ride I did not want, going to a place I feared and could not comprehend, not choosing, not understanding the cacophony of the absurd that was to be my life.

The next stop was the Scott's facility. It didn't appear quite as ominous as Jackson, but it was large, ugly, gray, with many rows of tall fencing topped with razor wire. We entered a back way and parked. Then we sat, not knowing why. Another road sign. Waiting to be told to stand and move, I sat alone in the van for about an hour before being escorted into the prison compound, my leg hurting, sharp pains becoming constant. Two other vehicles with women prisoners waited as well.

Later I learned we had arrived during Formal Count Time. Count Time occurs five times daily in the prisons. The inmates must be in their cells and the prison is placed on lockdown. The inmates must all be accounted for before normal operation resumes. No one comes in or out during these periods. Count Time takes priority, I was beginning to learn.

At noon, the transport officer walked up and knocked on the window. Curtly, he told me to get out. This was not easy for me with my injuries and a walker. I moved slowly and awkwardly. He accompanied me inside the forbidding gates. The officer motioned me to a chair where I sat down while he silently took off my chains.

He turned away from me without a word and left. It seemed so easy for this officer to make it clear that I was nothing to him. His delivery was complete, I was no different than a bag of groceries or a bucket of nails; the job was done and the fact that I was human was not significant to him. I remember feeling overwhelmingly sad and empty.

A female guard instructed me to change into a robe

and sit on a bench. I sat in a small room by myself surrounded by glass walls until the women from the other vans joined me.

The bleak walls, cracked ceilings, and dirty floors had a strange energy that immediately drained me. Suddenly I was as terrified of the officers as the rest of prison life. They appeared to relish their authority and take pleasure from diminishing others. Here I was prey, unable to run, hoping only to hide, entering a world I had never imagined. Little did I know how well acquainted I would become with those dark human traits.

With each clang of the prison doors I shuddered. My hair stood out. My broken middle-aged body stood out. My middle-class values and education stood out. And I somehow knew that this was a place where I must not stand out if I was to survive for seven years before I might go home again.

One life had ended, many more had been devastated. I was to blame.

CHAPTER FOUR

"Since the accident I have felt alone, abandoned, detached and frightened. I have gone through the judicial system unaware of what could happen to me and now I live each day in a horrible place surrounded by many horrible people. I have experienced new forms of fear, humiliation, and mental pain that I didn't even know existed."

– Patty Steele, Journal Entry, April 21, 2012.

My first day in prison was interminable. The intake area had unfinished, grey cinder block walls and hard cement floors. There was no daylight. It reminded me of a dark basement. I was given loose, drab clothing, mostly used, but imprinted with my new identity, 686898. At that moment I failed to even wonder who wore the clothes before me. Only later did I wonder what might have happened before they were issued to me.

The pants were dark blue with orange stripes down the side. The blouses were navy with bright orange yoke panels. Three other women arrived shortly after me and I watched them smile at each other and for a guard when taking their picture. I couldn't imagine smiling. When it was my turn to stand in front of the camera, I was crying uncontrollably. When the officer showed me the photo for my new identification card, I barely recognized myself. So tired and so old, the face in the picture was distorted with fear. The officer observed me looking at my photo as though I didn't know who I was seeing. She tried to convince me everything would be okay. But what could possibly be okay?

I was instructed to go with the other new arrivals to the health care facilities. I did not know why, and I was too afraid to ask. One of the women knew the location because she had been imprisoned in Scott's before. We all followed her out the back of the building.

Jan and Mel, as I came to know them, were kind. They offered to push me in a wheelchair while I sat with my lap piled high with our duffle bags of newly issued prison garb.

Krys, our red-headed guide, was skinny and unkempt. She had once been a model, but her drug addiction had drained her good looks. Now she spoke continually of needing her medications. Krys was detoxing and drug-sick, but lucky for us she remembered the way around the prison grounds.

Jan was an upbeat woman. She attempted to make light of our situation and tried to make me feel a little less frightened. Jan was in prison on a drug-related charge. The oldest of our group, besides me, was Mel. I later learned she attempted to kill her husband while high on pills. All of us were from northern Michigan and we moved slowly across the prison yard with me in the wheelchair.

The buildings surrounded a large center courtyard. Other prisoners were outside, walking and socializing, but no one acknowledged us. We entered another cinder block building known by the prisoners as "death care." I was soon to learn that in Michigan prisons it is extremely unlucky to be sick; care is elusive.

My leg pain was raging, but my fear was more overwhelming. In the lobby of Health Care, we sat for more than an hour, waiting, not knowing what to do and unwilling to ask a guard. We talked quietly among ourselves about our charges and how long we spent in our local jails before being transferred. Finally, an officer called Jan's name. One by one we were taken into examination rooms. The room I was placed in was dirty, unlike any medical facility I had ever been in. Pale yellow walls were covered with dirt marks and gouges. Tile floors and counters were littered with dirt, hair, and paper. A ripped examination table stood in the middle of the room. A used and wrinkled sheet of white paper covered a portion of the exam table. I found a small plastic chair in the corner of the room. I sat and waited.

A nurse gave me a tuberculosis shot and asked general medical health questions. I told her about the throbbing pain I was experiencing. She told me that the doctor must see me before I could get any pain medication. The earliest this might be was on Tuesday after the Memorial holiday weekend. That was four days away. I begged, telling her my papers stated I needed pain medication. But pain and humanity were not relevant here, I quickly understood I would have to do without.

The long day was over when we arrived at Cord A, otherwise known as Reception, Guidance, and Counseling. It was 10 p.m. and I was assigned a cell by myself on the upper level of the unit, a handicapped cell. The women who arrived with me were given cells on the lower level where they would be double-bunked. I was envious of the others who would not be alone.

In the darkness of my cell I listened to the sounds of this place, the distant clang of a door, or the bark of an angry voice, indistinct but for the tone. This was a different depth of aloneness. No one was coming to help me. No one was coming to comfort me. No one knew or cared about the pain, the sadness, or the engulfing fear.

*   *   *

A night officer explained to me that a prisoner by the name of Lea had suggested I be put in the handicapped accessible cell upstairs. This inmate recognized that I couldn't climb the stairs and would need an elevator. I learned later Lea had an ulterior motive. She thought I would be a good person to live next to her cell. Another woman was moved out of the handicapped cell so I could move in.

This was not Lea's first time in prison. She had spent fourteen years on her first time around. Lea knew how to use her influence with officers who remembered her from her past stay. She knew how to care for herself in prison, especially in this unit which housed all the new prisoners.

Lea appeared very pregnant; she had extra privileges due to her condition. Lea could come and go to the bathroom at almost any time. She could go down to the main level of the unit for ice water without asking permission. Lea used this freedom of movement to her advantage. She operated a store out of her cell supplying the new prisoners with items they longed for, especially cigarettes. She charged double the cost of the commissary, but the items were available upon request. This business kept Lea supplied with all the extras she desired.

Lea later told me she expected to be incarcerated for only a few months. She had returned to prison due to a parole violation. She anticipated having her baby during this time behind bars with Michigan Department of Corrections picking up the bill. Her sister would care for the baby until she was released.

Something about me gave Lea the impression that I would be a good neighbor. She wanted me next door to her. She sized me up quickly as a person who would never question her actions or snitch on her, and she was right. Perhaps she recognized my overwhelming fear and figured I needed to make friends and not trouble.

My first week in Scott Prison was spent with sleepless nights, softly crying so no one would hear. The pain in my leg never let up. Lying still made it worse. My bed consisted of an iron frame with a two-inch rock-hard mattress that had been used by many. The stiffness and bumps in the mattress offered no comfort, especially to my injuries. I got up often to walk during the night hoping it might bring a reprieve. After several days of sleeplessness, my fatigue caught up to me and I managed to fall asleep for short periods but found myself waking to my own frightened screams. My dreams were dark and terrifying. I was embarrassed the next morning when other women told me they heard me. I shared my fears with no one.

Even after sleepless nights, the mornings started early. At 6:30 a.m. the morning officer woke the prisoners. Over a loudspeaker she announced bathroom use. We were expected to hear and respond quickly. We filed to the bathroom, one cell at a time, and then dressed for breakfast.

For a while I couldn't comprehend many of the garbled instructions over the loudspeaker. Understanding the pronunciations from different races and ethnic backgrounds was an embarrassing challenge for me. I grew up in Detroit but lived in a predominately white neighborhood. I later moved to northern Michigan and attended a primarily white college. My work experience was with white people. I struggled to understand the dialects and slang I was hearing, and this posed a problem for me, but I was afraid of letting others know. Instead, I often found myself foolishly nodding my head affirmatively when I had no clue what someone said to me. I now lived with criminals from all backgrounds and ethnicities, and clearly did not know how to make it in this environment. I did not know if I would ever fit in or ever feel safe.

*   *   *

Prison was monotony and tightly enforced schedules. Loud voices barked orders over speakers and the guards scowled. There were so many rules to learn, the loss of identity, powerlessness, and endless hours of boredom. Cell doors were kept closed at all times. We could not leave our cells without permission; there was no standing in the doorways or communicating with other prisoners while in our cells. It was against the rules to gaze out the small window on the door of my cell to watch the activity in the unit. There was no asking to use the bathroom during shift changes or Count Times.

Lea arranged for a prisoner to get my meals to me from the main level. In Cord A, the new inmates were not allowed to interact with general prison population, so meals were brought from what was called the chow hall to our unit.

Lea took it upon herself to choose Christy, a young black woman, to be my helper. She delivered my meals to me three times a day. On the few occasions I was expected to leave the unit, Christy pushed me in a wheelchair. Lea assured me Christy was free of diseases when telling me she would be my designated aid. I know that Lea meant this piece of information to be comforting, but in truth it made me fear the presence of diseases among the other prisoners, and how much of the population was afflicted.

Christy was happy to get out of her cell whenever she could. I soon recognized she was also an assistant to Lea for her store business. I cared nothing about the commerce that was going on around me. I understood Lea was taking care of her and I was just grateful for her kind help.

Shower time began after breakfast. Again, cell by cell, we were allowed ten minutes to shower and brush teeth. There was a bathroom on both ends of our hallway with three toilet stalls, three sinks, and one shower. These bathrooms were never clean. My cell was the second one away from the bathroom, so I had to be ready to shower quickly after breakfast. We were expected to be in our robes and shower shoes, quickly move to the shower when it was our turn, and then get dressed in our cells.

Nudity was not recommended as it was taken as a signal of homosexuality, which was rampant, although not condoned by the prison. There was a phrase inside, "Gay for the stay, straight at the gate." Many women for many different reasons experimented with their sexuality while in prison.

I had no interest in a homosexual relationship and no knowledge of how to communicate this effectively. I was not interested in prison sex games. I was a handicapped alcoholic, but also a slim woman with long blond hair.

I found myself alone in the bathroom one morning with one other inmate. She was wearing a robe but holding it open to dry herself under a hand dryer. She turned toward me and flashed her naked body at me with a wickedly inviting smile. I looked away with embarrassment and left quickly. I had no clue how to react. After that I became even more wary of everyone's intention. My normal was not the same as the other prisoners. I was offended and reactive to behaviors that others found insignificant, of no importance. That included unwanted advances.

Count Time occurred twice during daytime hours, after breakfast and again at 4 p.m. During Count Time all prisoners were required to be in their cells, visible on their bunks, with their doors secured and identification in the window of the door. Anyone out of compliance risked a major ticket violation. Multiple major tickets resulted in segregation and a higher security level. They could impact future requests for parole.

The officers went cell-by-cell accounting for every prisoner. Once the Control Center confirmed total headcount, Count Time ended. Usually it took thirty or forty minutes, but sometimes it took hours. If an officer reported an incorrect head count, the total prison count would be off, and the count would have to be retaken until every prisoner was accounted for. An officer could receive a formal demerit in their employment record for an inaccurate count, so they took it seriously.

On my second morning in the Scott Prison, I learned the seriousness of Count Time rules. I'd fallen asleep on my bunk after showering without securing my door tightly. Officer Brown, a commanding and fearsome officer, woke me threatening to give me a ticket for not adhering to count rules. I realized quickly my fate was in the hands of others. Luckily, she only issued me a sanction, which was less severe than a major ticket violation and did not go on any permanent record.

The sanction restricted me to my cell for the next three days. I was permitted only to leave to use the bathroom. This meant I could not take part in the one hour of nightly freedom within the unit that lasted from 7:30 p.m. to 8:30 p.m. for the upper level prisoners. During this hour some used the phone, others watched TV or played cards, and many spent the time picking books from the main floor library to read during the long days.

Through the haze of my pain I adapted to a world that made little sense to me, lining up, waiting for permission to move, following the schedule, watching any sense of my personal identity fade away, becoming Michigan Prisoner #686898.

Lunch was scheduled at 11 a.m. Prisoners who had pre-arranged activities usually were scheduled to do them in the afternoon. Cord A was the intake section of the prison. It was here that security assessments, testing, and informational groups were held. The prison required new inmates to be informed about AIDS, Hepatitis B and C, and the correction department's sexual conduct policy.

The 4 p.m. count was followed by chow or dinner. The evenings consisted of our one-hour free time with other inmates and being locked up the rest of the night. When it was the upper level's turn for free time, I gladly rode the elevator down hoping to interact with some of the women and get books to fill the long hours. Loneliness was a constant companion. Often, I stood in my door watching out the small oblong window and wondering about the women I saw who lived downstairs. I was careful to avoid being detected by the officers.

I longed to call home and hear familiar voices, but there was a complex process for phone privileges which included acquiring a phone pin and having the prison approve your phone list. We were required to list the names and their numbers for phone use. Approval took time so I was unable to speak to my family for a month. I wondered if they missed me, I wondered if they were afraid for me. I wondered if they were pleased I was gone.

Each day I spent many hours looking out the one exterior window in my cell where I could see the outside. The window was small and had bars on it that restricted the view. It overlooked the prison yards. I watched hundreds of women come and go to the yard for exercise and fresh air throughout the day.

One group of women especially fascinated me. These women were allowed to use the whole prison yard by themselves in the morning, but in the evening when other prisoners were present, they were secluded in a small fenced area. They obviously were barred from interacting with the rest of the prison population. I learned these women were in Level Four security with only one level higher. Level Five was reserved for people in total segregation twenty-four hours continually.

The Level Four women I watched out my tiny window included those considered problem prisoners, dangerous, as well as new arrivals believed threatening to general population due to their long length of sentence and the seriousness of their charge. I soon discovered that anyone with a sentence of six years or more was placed in Level Four before joining the general population.

* * *

On May 30, six days after arriving in prison, I turned forty-nine years old. My birthday always seemed special, with family and friends gathering to celebrate during Memorial Day weekend. I told no one of my birthday until the day was almost over and remained stuck in thoughts of my own pain and loneliness. Finally, I reached out.

From the door of my cell I spoke to Helen, the woman in the next handicapped cell. She was a comforting presence and I somehow knew she would understand my loneliness. Helen was in a wheelchair due to the loss of one leg. A heavy-set black woman in her fifties, she had been in prison four times. She swore this time was her last. A drug addict, she had lost her leg from using tainted drugs and lamented the repeated loss of her freedom.

Helen prayed a lot and read her Bible throughout the day. She was soft-spoken and I liked her, none of which made sense when I considered her life of addiction and criminal behaviors. Somehow my conversations with Helen spurred me to more deeply consider how substance abuse leads to the destruction of so many lives, including my own.

On this night, I risked a sanction from the guards for speaking. I had no doubt that if they overheard the conversation between cells we would be reprimanded and given a punishment. I was scared, but I was desperate to connect. I whispered from behind the bars in the darkness as quietly as I could sharing with Helen that it was my birthday. In response, she told me of her faith in God's love and forgiveness.

But I could no longer feel God's presence in my life. My God had once brought me comfort, but now there was none. I felt only forgotten. I was now a caged animal, less than human, my life held no decent future that I could see. My past and any good I may have done were erased by all my sins. All that was gone, the steel door and bars on the window were real. The garbled announcements, the strident commands, and the rigid schedule were real.

*   *   *

June of 2008 was unbearably hot. The temperatures outside were in the 90s and it was even warmer in the cells. The prisoners' units had no air conditioning and the only fans were located at the officer's desk. The stagnant heat went on for weeks; women were fainting and becoming sick. Most of us were too fearful to complain to the officers. We understood that our welfare was not important to them. However, after repeated episodes of women experiencing heat stroke, fans finally appeared for the inmates. They were placed in the hallways outside our cells. We were allowed to crack our doors slightly during the day for relief.

I spent most of those days lying on my bed reading and wondering about home. My children were foremost in my thoughts. Without access to phone calls, I wrote letters to my kids in which I told them nothing of what prison was truly like. Instead, I made up jokes about how I had learned to roll big, fat cigarettes and lie to the guards. My leg continued to keep me up during the night. In the morning I got in line for the bathroom completely exhausted. For me, with my limited ability to walk, there was no exercise beyond using my walker to move in small circles in the cell. I had no chance to get out into the fresh air.

Health Care refused to see me even after an officer reported my discomfort. I began to realize I was in pain not only from the injury, but I was detoxing from the opiate medication that was abruptly discontinued. Detoxing intensified the pain; my body was still detoxing from my years of alcoholism. As I tried to figure out how to live this new life, each day I felt horrible, unsteady, mentally fogged.

My assessment period in Cord A lasted forty-five days. In July, two nights before I was moved out of the unit, an officer who I'd never seen before in our unit asked to speak with me as I made my way to the elevator. I was taking my nightly cup of ice water up to my cell moving slowly with my walker. Other prisoners were already in their cells.

This officer asked me why I was in prison. I told her of the accident and my alcoholism. She listened and then told me I was different from other prisoners. She said I would get through my years and go home, never to return. She was compassionate and sympathetic. She seemed to understand my worries of surviving the next seven years.

For a moment we stood silently together and then the officer told me that her own child was killed by a drunk driver. At that moment I was completely confused about the kindness she was showing me. All I could think of was the sorrow she must have endured losing a child to a drunk driver. She saw my bewilderment. She shared with me her years working in the prison helped her understand that the driver who killed her son had not intended for the accident to happen.

I felt her forgiveness in that moment. I went back to my cell and thought about our conversation throughout the night. I intended to thank this woman as soon as I saw her again and tell her how her how much her words had meant to me. But she wasn't there the next night or the following night.

Two days later I learned that I was being moved to Cord B, Level Four security. My days in Registration, Guidance, and Counseling were up and a bed was available for me in this new unit. No one warned me that my crime would place me with those dangerous female prisoners. I never considered that a middle-aged white woman with a walker, untreated for pain and barely able to get through each day, might somehow be placed among a feared and heavily restricted group. This was the group I had watched from my cell window, the women kept segregated from the rest of the prison's population.

"Steele, pack up and be ready to move," came the garbled order over the intercom.

CHAPTER FIVE

"I'm 49 years old and in prison. If I'd been allowed to stay home between my guilty verdict and sentencing, I would have finally figured out how to take my life. That would have been easier than knowing prison was my future. My family would hurt, but life goes on. Time heals wounds."

– Patty Steele, Journal Entry, 2008.

The officer at the desk looked me up and down but said little. Basic courtesies are seldom exchanged in prison. The Level Four female officer pointed toward the elevator and told me I was assigned downstairs to Cord B, Cell 62. No help was offered.

There was no opportunity to say goodbye to Lea, Christy, or Helen. I struggled getting to the elevator, shuffling my walker and dragging my faded duffel bag. I understood no one was going to volunteer to help me. Courtesy is not a tool inside prison walls, friendliness is viewed with suspicion. Manipulation is rampant, based not on social skills but rather on fear and pain in the halls of punishment.

With difficulty, I maneuvered my duffle bag and walker inside the elevator. It operated differently than the one in

Cord A and I felt awkward standing alone fumbling with the buttons, not sure how to proceed. Finally, I figured it out and began my descent down to high security prison life.

Managing new challenges in prison is different from living in the outside world where you can seek out advice, reach for a tool, look at a video, or ask someone for help. Asking for help is weakness in a place where weakness makes you vulnerable. In some ways I was prepared for this aspect of prison since in my own life I'd hidden my fears and hurts for so long, not knowing how to ask for help.

On the lower level the elevator opened to two large handicapped cells on my left, a sitting area of three tables and chairs on my right, and a bathroom straight ahead. Cell 62 was past the bathroom, to the right and halfway down the hallway. I no longer had a handicapped cell. Instead, I now shared a regular cell with a roommate or bunkie. Her name was Alice.

Alice kindly offered to help me with my bag and then left the cell so I could get settled. Our cell was the size of a large closet. Long ago it had been painted white, now it showed signs of the many who had lived there. Against the back wall there was an iron bunk bed with a thin, bare mattress pad on the bottom for me. On each side of the cell, against the cinder block walls, stood a double metal locker, a metal desk with a chair, and a bulletin board positioned over each desk. The bulletin board was for family pictures and mementos. All other possessions were expected to be stored in the locker or under the desk unless in use. Only a Bible and a glass of water were allowed on the desk; nothing could be taped to the walls. Sanctions were given for rooms out of order. This cell was neat, it had no strong odors and I was happy to know I had a clean roommate.

Later that day, Alice shared with me some parts of her personal story. She was in her early thirties and in prison for life. Alice had no chance of parole. She entered Scott Prison a few months before me and before that she spent close to a year in a county jail. She arrived in Cord B only a couple months before, but long enough to have learned much about prison life. Alice had friends in this unit and was adjusting.

Alice looked young, was pretty with long red hair. I struggled to imagine what she could possibly have done to receive life in prison. The same was true with many of the women I was to meet. Having a bunkie was going to be a change, but I welcomed it. I hoped not to feel as lonely having someone to talk with. I also was relieved Alice was white.

This sounds horrible, but I had already witnessed many women in prison fighting over racial issues that I did not understand or know how to handle. Arguments erupted when a bunkie's hair landed on the other's bunk. White women were accused of having hair that floated throughout the cell. Black women were accused of not washing their hair often enough resulting in bad odors.

Racial tension was real in prison and women were characterized by their race. I observed black women often presented themselves as loud and aggressive. It was as if they were saying; "Do not challenge me." White women tended to be more passive, which was often viewed as a weakness by black prisoners. I knew I'd have to quickly develop my own voice, learn how to confront people and not be steamrolled by prisoners or guards. A weak person is at risk in prison. Regardless of race, if a weak woman is in the wrong place at the wrong time, she is vulnerable.

The respect of other prisoners is a form of protection and safety in that world.

Once, my life included many acts of gentleness. But I'd destroyed that life along with my marriage, my health, and my relationships with my children.

My phone list was finally approved, and I could call my children during free time out of the cell. The calls from prison were expensive and reaching them by phone was not always possible. I told them I was fine when we spoke. Nothing about my world made sense to me. But hiding my fears was nothing new.

*   *   *

Alice tried to make me feel comfortable. She shared some luxuries that were not allowed in Cord A. She gave me tweezers, fingernail clippers, and a razor bought from commissary. My fingernails were like claws. They had always grown fast and during my time in Cord A they became grotesquely long. I didn't break them off because I had nothing to file them smoothly. My face was a mess. Without proper tools or any decent place to care for myself, I dug at my chin with a pen cap to remove the occasional unwanted facial hairs. To do this, I positioned the tail of a pen cap next to my skin and the hair and pulled. Sometimes it worked, others took many attempts and left my face scratched from the plastic of the cap. My chin was pocked with scabs.

I was excited to shave, though I had never seen such a flimsy razor. It had a single blade that was so thin it could be folded in half. Yet I was grateful. My legs and underarms were hairy messes making me feel dirty and less feminine. I was happy to shave no matter the many little cuts I received on my newly hairless skin.

Lack of self-care can be terribly embarrassing for female prisoners as some grow mustaches and beards. Newly arrived inmates could not yet order the basic supplies available to most prisoners, giving them more opportunity for degradation. Prisoners and staff cruelly ridiculed their appearance and these verbal attacks were demeaning and humiliating. For me, though I did not have excess body hair, shaving made me feel more respectable and human.

* * *

Level Four housed the inmates whose crimes were most serious, along with those whose behaviors made them a greater danger to the guards or inmates. Some were mentally ill, and I learned to cautiously avoid them. Others were just reactive, easily angered, and more likely to be aggressive. Arguing with guards, yelling or screaming resulted in punishments. Women who reacted in this manner were sanctioned to their cells for days, their issues ignored. Those who responded with hostility found themselves handcuffed and escorted to segregation for an undetermined time. These aggressive interactions frightened me. My forty-nine-year old damaged body, with its constant nagging pain, was poorly equipped to handle physical violence. And then there was the emotional aspect of degrading behavior unfamiliar to me. I wasn't good at it and just wanted to hide from it.

Often prisoners had real concerns about living conditions, treatment by the guards, and health issues. Many women in Level Four only knew how to express concerns by flying into anger and aggression. The results were predictable, leading to more yelling, brief flurries of violence, guards swarming with handcuffs, unit lockdowns, and isolation for punishment. It always led to the same poor results, but this fruitless behavior continued no matter the lack of positive outcomes. We live with patterns in our lives, the behaviors we know, the responses we have learned. It made no sense to me, but something about observing these patterns reminded me of my own life before my accident on the road near Interlochen.

My own pain continued to plague me. In my forty-five days in Registration, Guidance, and Counseling I was unable to see a doctor. Now in Level Four the staff continued to ignore my requests.

Alice began my education regarding the prison grievance system. This system was the only recourse for prisoners in most instances. A vast majority of complaints were discarded by the prison based upon minor technicalities. Staff did all they could possibly do to avoid addressing the complaints of the women.

A prisoner had to file a timely and precisely written grievance to have a review challenging a specific treatment or lack of one. The prisoner had to prove some action or inaction caused harm, identify the specific prison policy that was violated, and supply evidence to prove how it happened.

Most inmates failed to file grievances that were clear, to the point, and backed by policy within the allotted time. The prison employed staff whose only job was to review grievances for process errors. They did not hesitate to deny them even if these concerns were urgent and undeniably true.

Grievances found to be accurate and irrefutable, generally represented admission of a wrongdoing by the prison or its staff. The officers and the administration did not appreciate being in the wrong. They protected each other at all costs. When a grievance involving staff was investigated, we knew their colleagues would willingly lie for them. A prisoner had to possess concrete evidence such as actions or words caught on camera, written documentation, or unassailable collaboration to have the prison take some action on their behalf.

Few grievances were won by prisoners, but if they were, it was only after a long process taking months and the filing of appeals. Yet, successful grievances could result in better food in the chow hall, cleaning supplies for the living units, health care, a return to the general prison population from segregation, and on occasion, the disciplining of a guard.

When I learned I had access to the Scott Prison Law Library, I was ready to explore prison policies and legal safeguards. Spending time there offered a respite. The walls were wood, and the floors were carpeted. There were books, not romance novels or self-help tomes, but shelves of quiet strength. Being in the Law Library was an escape from the chaos, a place of reason and learning. Later the library would become my steady friend.

* * *

My many attempts to get help for my chronic leg pain were summarily rejected. In the Law Library I learned that this rejection without consideration was a violation of prison policy. Health Care's refusal to give me an appointment could be dealt with through the grievance system.

A few weeks after arriving in Level Four, I was about to

put my first Health Care grievance into the prison mail system when I was approached by a superior officer, Captain Martin. He was a tall, lean man with graying hair at the temples and a kind face. He wore blue jeans and a sports coat. I had never seen him before, but I knew he was the assistant to the warden.

I was surprised to see Captain Martin approaching me. He spotted the grievance packet in my hand and noticed my walker along with my inability to use my right leg. He asked with concern about the problems I was experiencing. I explained my injuries and the many requests to officers in the unit as well as to Health Care for help. I explained that all had gone unanswered.

Captain Martin offered me his help. He asked me to wait and give him a chance to address the problem personally. He said he would make sure Health Care scheduled an appointment with me soon. I was amazed that he offered his assistance. I felt extremely lucky that he was willing to go out of his way for me. Even though he was trying to avoid my filing a grievance, it was also an act of consideration, not the norm for prison staff behavior.

Ignoring physical, emotional, and spiritual pain is the well-established norm in prison. These norms resist even the intervention of the top brass. Captain Martin visited Health Care daily for over a week until I was placed on what is known as a call out for an appointment. A call out is an official document, a piece of paper, allowing a prisoner to move on the prison grounds at an appointed time to another location. The call outs were printed nightly and delivered to the inmate's cell during the early morning hours while most were sleeping. The prisoner must carry the call out slip as proof of permission to move about the grounds. Many prisoners had multiple call outs daily for activities such as receiving daily medications. Other inmates had daily or occasional call outs for work, school, the gym, Alcoholic Anonymous, Health Care, or the Law Library.

Captain Martin made no progress with Health Care initially but didn't give up. He kept me informed of his progress (or lack of) by coming to my unit or catching me in the chow hall. Even as a ranking prison official, he had limited authority over the Health Care operations. Those functions were run by private companies to save costs. I gradually learned how many operations in prison involved cost-saving measures.

A few months before I arrived at Scott Prison, a correction officer was shot by a fellow officer after work at a gas station across the street from the prison. Tension between the two officers was known by staff and administration but not handled. Proactivity is not the norm in American prisons, but a public mess invites scrutiny and Captain Martin and Warden Washington were brought in to be the clean-up team.

I was finally scheduled to see a doctor. Two months after my first day in prison, a doctor wrote me a prescription for Ultram, a mild pain reliever. She was a Korean woman whose English was broken and difficult to understand. She said it was the only pain reliever she could prescribe without a formal assessment by Lansing officials. Medications of all sorts, especially narcotics, were limited and strictly reviewed. These rules defended against abuse and black-market sales while cutting costs. Upon arrival at prison, inmates on prescriptions were often refused their medication as I was or switched to a cheaper substitute medication. This pattern was part of the reason why so many physical and mental health issues were intensified within the prison walls.

Call outs became part of my daily routine. Each day I reported to Health Care between 7 a.m. and 8 a.m., whenever medications were announced for Level Four. I went again about noon and before nightly lockdown. Standing in a long line of prisoners, I waited while the nurse distributed medications through a small exterior window in the Health Care building. Upon reaching the window, I gave her my name and my prison identification number before she gave me my pill. She watched me as I swallowed it and there was no banter. I understood the precautions and I was becoming accustomed to the lack of trust and constant indignities.

With the medication, I could bear some weight on my right leg and walk with less pain. Best of all, I could finally sleep for a few hours at a time.

* * *

Level Four inmates had their meals in the chow hall at a separate time from the general population. The meals at Scott were better than the food in the county jail and I finally found my appetite. There were fresh fruits and vegetables daily, the main dishes contained real meat and the kitchen staff was proud of their efforts. I began to gain unwanted weight with my own injuries limiting my movement along with the monotonous daily prison routine.

Mel, who I'd met my first day at Scott's, was already in Level Four when I arrived. She was willing to walk with me for meals and act as my aid. She carried my food tray and sat with me. Most afternoons we encountered an officer on the walkway who took pleasure in demeaning women on their way to and from the chow hall. He was a large black man who regularly confronted Mel for being with me on my slow walk. He accused her of dawdling.

Prisoners were not supposed to loiter on the walkways. But this guard's behavior was an unnecessary abuse of his power. He was entertaining himself by making us cower. After many days of this, I decided to speak up and tell him what he already knew, that Mel was acting as an aid for me. I didn't want her continually assaulted by his words for helping me, but I feared I would be his next target. I wasn't confrontational when responding to his berating tone. Most prisoners either silently submit to authority or became inflamed. Common reactions were either fight or flight in prison.

A few days after I defended Mel, the officer pulled me aside as we were walking back from lunch. I was nervous and afraid of what he might say or do. He called me by name, which worried me more, and asked why I was in prison. I told him the truth. I realized he probably already knew, as the information was easily available to the guards. The officer didn't have much else to say to me and let me go. Thankful, I felt I had just dodged a bullet.

A few days after our conversation on the walkway, the same officer approached me again. This time he wanted to talk. He shared with me a personal story of an incident that had occurred several years earlier. He was driving close to home and he was drunk. He lived with his mother. He hit something in the dark, he didn't know what it was, but believed it could have been a person.

Rather than stop he became afraid, left the scene, and drove home. His mother convinced him, a grown man, to return to the scene. A person was hit, but not badly hurt. In the end, there were no repercussions and he was thankful. He knew he could have faced charges and described the panic he had felt. Most of all he was relieved that he did not have to live with unanswered questions for the rest of his life.

I'm not sure why this officer chose to share his story with me. He continued to be an abusive prick who bullied women on the walkway, but sometimes he'd see me and offer the smallest nod of acknowledgement.

* * *

The lower bunk I occupied in cell 62 had previously been the home of a woman named Gem. She was released after many years at Scott's facility, but Gem must have been a problem prisoner as she had resided in Level Four before leaving. Alice informed me that Gem shared her plans to file a lawsuit against a male officer who was still employed at Scott's facility after her release, accusing this officer of fathering her 14-year-old son. There was no question of Gem becoming pregnant while in prison, only of the parentage. Interestingly, this officer's wife was our regular morning officer in Level Four.

The morning officer was a no-nonsense guard, but fair. She was stern and ran a tight ship when on duty. I would often see her husband in the educational building when I visited the Law Library. He was soft-spoken and a gentleman, opening the door for me as I shuffled along on my walker. He helped me on the elevator.

In 2009, the Michigan Courts reached a settlement of $100 million dollars for approximately five hundred women who claimed sexual assault, abuse, and sexual harassment by the male staff of The Michigan Department of Corrections. This is known as the Neal Suit named for one of the women who initiated it.

Payments to the prisoners were made over a five-year period. During my time in prison, I met many female prisoners who received money from the state. Some payments were in the hundreds of thousands; some were in the millions. There were also women I met, who like Gem, had not become part of the Neal Suit and planned to sue upon release. One of the consequences of the lawsuit was that a few prisoners possessed lots of money. Some used their wealth to pay for illicit drugs which were reportedly supplied by staff. According to the prison grapevine, cocaine could be had for a five hundred dollar minimum.

* * *

It took a few months before I learned more about Alice's story. In prison, most women are cautious about sharing too much information. Painful truths, lies, and half-lies can be used to bully and intimidate. Guilt and shame are constant companions behind bars, easily roused by a few malicious words.

My own pattern of hiding my alcoholism and addictive behaviors made it easy to understand the reticence to share. Not yet understanding or trusting the strange landscape of a women's prison made me even more wary. Most of the time I kept my thoughts and memories to myself. My shame was my own, not to be shared like a sleazy reality show. It helped that my age and background stood out. I was atypical and few inmates found satisfaction in meddling in my past. For me, it was a quiet and lonely existence. I craved understanding, friendship, touch, and forgiveness, but I could not yet imagine any of these becoming partners again in my life.

In the safety of our cell, Alice gradually decided she could trust me. The desire to share her story outweighed her fear of judgement and betrayal. She was a rebellious adolescent, her mother struggled to control her. Alice married young and was quickly unhappy. Drugs became her entertainment and then escape.

Alice had a baby, but her addiction won out over her husband and young son. She was drawn to the wilder side where drugs were plentiful. She became a self-described dancer, a stripper and a party girl. On the day of her crime, Alice had taken her boyfriend to an acquaintance's mobile home. They needed money for drugs and this man, a friend, gave her money in the past. This time, instead of asking they intended to rob him. During the robbery the boyfriend shot the man dead while Alice stood by.

Alice sincerely did not understand how her life ended up this way. She chose risky behaviors that were exciting for her not knowing where they might lead. After a while, all of Alice's energies went into surviving as a young drug addict on the streets. Now she lived the consequences, life in prison. Alice would never know freedom again.

It occurred to me that Alice was just not facing reality. It was too painful, and she couldn't face the reality that she chose the drugs, left her child, ran with drug dealers, and stood by while a man was murdered. For a moment I judged her and found her guilty, then it hit me like a punch in the belly. I chose to drink and drive and brought pain to my family and the Jones family. It was not any different.

There is so much sadness dwelling on a future that is

bleak. My bunkie learned to avoid thinking about the future and the past. It is easier to just live in the minute, not looking forward or backward, not pondering responsibility and judgement. This is often the mindset of long term survival in prison. I practiced this coping skill as an alcoholic. It simply hurts too much to reflect upon all the moments and opportunities lost.

*   *   *

As the months went on, Alice found a source for pills and was high a lot. She began a gay relationship with a woman named Karr. Alice told me she was heterosexual, but that no longer seemed to matter. If she wanted a relationship to call her own it would be with another woman. Alice had many gay relationships I witnessed during my seven years. There was always prison gossip about who was "hooking up." Girlfriends were seen sitting together in the units or in the yard. Sex took place in cells, bathrooms, and sometimes publicly in the yard. Some prisoners were discreet, while others enjoyed the attention of others watching.

Karr and Alice held a mock wedding ceremony in the halls of Level Four and proclaimed themselves married. They made childish rings and exchanged them. They held hands when out of view of the officers. I asked no questions; I didn't want to know. I understood that being gay was natural for some, but this was not a natural situation and I did not want to be witness. I understood Alice wanted to feel special. Feeling good does not come easily in prison. Like many of my reactions to prison life, I looked the other way.

In our cell, Alice and I occasionally had conversations

about her feeling confused and possibly mistaking dangerous prison games for real life. Her behaviors in prison were rapidly becoming increasingly risky, reflecting her lack of hope for the future. It worried me that she would be physically hurt by another prisoner or confined to long-term segregation. As her drug use increased, she became a difficult cellmate. She was no longer content unless high. Getting her pills was costing her more money than she had. She became irritable and sick when the pills were withheld by her supplier for lack of funds. In prison, no one was going to feel sorry for Alice.

Alice hated when her commissary from the prison store arrived every two weeks. She generally owed everything she received from the commissary for her drugs. Often, she was short and called her mother for extra funds. Her mother had little money and could seldom help. Alice became angry at her mother and would yell at her during phone conversations, accuse her mother of not caring. Eventually Alice's mother stopped visiting and accepted fewer of her calls. Alice's self-destructive and addictive behavior was controlling her life now in prison and making her increasingly miserable every day.

In our cell our relationship became strained; I was upset, yet I could sympathize. Alice felt nothing could hurt her more than life already had. Her behavior no longer mattered. She escaped mentally with drugs. It seemed that her spirit was somehow diminishing.

I watched in silence and thought of my own addiction. I thought of my personal loss of control, my battles to regain a life worth living, and my own failures to succeed no matter how much I wanted something better.

*   *   *

I was struck by the presence and amount of illegal drug use in prison by inmates. The two main sources were prisoners' prescribed medications and officers supplying illicit drugs. Prison officials contended that visitors brought drugs into the prison, but in my experience, this was rarely true.

Prisoners who were prescribed narcotics or any other strong medications must visit Health Care to obtain them. In prison, this is known as medlines. Some prisoners were known to cheek their medications or hide them in their cheek rather than swallow them, and later sell them. The Health Care personnel were instructed to watch for this practice, but it was difficult to detect. Inmates are good at deception.

Prisoners found selling their medications or hiding them in their cells were written major tickets for substance abuse. They were taken into custody and placed in segregation, often for long periods of time.

Some officers brought drugs, cigarettes, and other contraband into the prison for the right amount of money. Officers were frisked daily as they entered the prison compound, but this was done with little vigilance by their peers. Corrections officers have a brotherhood. Even if they don't like or condone a colleague's actions, they support each other by looking away.

Once, after cigarettes were banned in the prison, I shared a contraband cigarette that cost ten dollars bought by Mel. Sometimes I saw marijuana being smoked on the prison grounds and I heard of crack cocaine being available. And, as I found less need for my Ultram, I sold some of it to another woman in my unit. This allowed me extra commissary items which the woman bought for me, a common practice although a major violation of the rules.

One day, I was outside of Cord B walking to the yard. An inmate named Brenda was assigned to care for her unit's gardens. She was working in the front of the building which was adjacent to the prisoner's walkways. Many varieties of flowers were in bloom. I saw her sitting on a retaining wall of a flower bed taking a break. Cigarettes had not been banned at this time and Brenda appeared to be smoking one. I looked at her and realized she was smoking something, but the way she inhaled it did not look like a cigarette to me. I asked her about it, and she laughed gloriously. She asked me if the gardens smelled good and then told me she found smoking pot openly in the gardens much safer than hiding in the unit. I remember thinking she was smarter than most. Over the years when I saw Brenda I would ask, "How are your gardens?" And we laughed thinking of that moment.

* * *

While in Level Four, I witnessed one prisoner being taken by ambulance to the hospital on many occasions. Heddie sold her epilepsy medication for commissary goods. While it was not unusual to see prisoners on the grounds having epileptic seizures, Heddie's seizures were severe. Whenever Heddie had a particularly intense seizure, Health Care staff was called to the unit. The unit was locked down and she was evaluated. Her seizures could go on for hours and she was frequently difficult to wake afterward. If a decision was made to take Heddie to the hospital, an ambulance was called. The whole compound was placed on lockdown while the ambulance came and went from the grounds.

None of this happened quickly. The prison medical staff arrived unhurriedly, and an ambulance was called only when Health Care believed her condition was life threatening. Handcuffs and leg restraints were placed on Heddie as she lay unconscious. She was lifted onto a gurney and strapped down. No escape precaution was too small for a convicted criminal, no matter their physical condition. The prison returned once again to normal operations only when the ambulance was outside the prison gates.

Heddie always returned, although sometimes it took several days. I never knew her to stop selling her medication. Her commissary items were her special comforts and she could not afford them on her own. A few candies, some cookies, and maybe some lotion for her cracked dry skin were more important than her health or her life.

CHAPTER SIX

"I realize now my family was dysfunctional. Drinking and our inability to communicate left us without healthy coping mechanisms. What I learned as a child I carried into my adult life."

– Patty Steele, Journal Entry, 2010.

The days were long and lonely in prison, dragging into months. It began to feel normal being ordered to wake, use the bathroom, eat, go outside, and speak or not. Each day I felt unsafe, watching for the outbreaks of viciousness that might occur, looking for that look or gesture that preceded genuine acts of violence. I'd learned to avoid eye contact with the guards and to endure endless verbal humiliations. I was learning the prison rules for playing it safe. Life in prison became my new normal. I was an insignificant being in a place where no one could save me.

In prison, living in the past or future is both dangerous and painful. It is painful because there are so many regrets to consider. It is dangerous because you need to be vigilant, attentive to signs of trouble from other prisoners or from the guards. Better to live in the moment, alert to danger, following the schedule, undistracted by daydreams and nightmares. Easier said than done. My thoughts often drifted to the people and places that were no longer present in my life.

I began to wonder if I had more in common with the other prisoners than I realized. The amenities and opportunities of my old life were now gone. No more dressing up for a special evening, no more running up to the store for a treat or another bottle. The small diversions, sitting by a lake, some music, a walk in the woods, a silly conversation, were all gone. The patterns of life were so completely different now, so consistently demeaning, and so completely outside of my control.

From a distance, my old life looked different. The life I once believed to be gratifying was starting to look shallow. It was obvious that many of my relationships lacked honesty and kindness. Clearly, they were lacking the promise of commitment through difficult times, because amid these difficult times I was so alone. Each morning waking to the garbled loudspeaker, or during the long nights when pain kept me awake, or sometimes when waiting in a line of women in the long corridors of our unit, I wondered how I got here.

There was no obvious abuse or neglect in our home while growing up. From the outside my family appeared a large and ambitious bunch. My parents sent us to good Catholic schools and encouraged academic and non-academic achievements. Our neighborhood was safe, the streets were lined with over-arching trees, our home was large. Friends and opportunities were plentiful. It was what I knew, I thought this life and my family were normal.

The bad times usually revolved around my parents' drinking. As kids, we did not speak of their relationship problems or their excessive drinking. We didn't speak of their endless arguments or the control my father held tightly over all of us. Both of my parents liked their nightly cocktails, though seldom together. My mother began openly drinking while preparing dinner.

While dinner cooked, my mother often relaxed with a drink in our living room. I'd watch her drinking alone and listening to romantic 1940s music on the stereo. She was companionless. My parents had clear roles as provider and homemaker, but they seldom acted in a loving way toward each other. My father returned home from his work day just in time for dinner. He joined the family already at the dinner table with a drink in hand. I can picture him giving my mother a peck on the cheek before taking his seat at the far end of the table. Most nights she would turn her cheek away from his gesture.

Depending upon the amount of alcohol they consumed, dinner table conversation could be more than unkind. I often thought we should tape these exchanges and play them back for them later. In my child's eyes, I believed they did not recognize the cruel and underhanded words they exchanged. Their fights were about money, kids, and infidelity. They held on to resentments. We observed these arguments as part of the family dinner routine. If friends or neighbors joined our family for a meal or an evening, the arguments went underground, hidden except for a poisoned barb that could be explained as a joke, or a killing glance not intended to be noticed by others outside the family.

My father was known in the family to be unfaithful to my mother. He told me once as an adult that "if you don't get it at home, you find it elsewhere." My mother was consistently wounded by my father's words and actions and he was stung by her sharp verbal attacks and coldness. As smart as they were, they never knew how to communicate with one another. With only respect for each other's talents, they were unable to create a marriage of trust and intimacy. Difficulty with trust became a learned pattern throughout our family.

My parents were from different backgrounds. They both lived through the Depression as teenagers and young adults. My mother grew up in a home of privilege and secrets. She was the daughter of one of the founders of the former A&P grocery store chain. She was also abused by her grandfather and told by her mother to keep this secret to herself so that her father and the rest of the world would not know. This betrayal destroyed any possibility of being a trusting person throughout her life.

After years of living a life with beautiful clothes, good schools, and chauffeured automobiles, her father died of alcoholism when she was twenty. Her family was left with a mess of debts and a sudden change of fortune.

My father was raised in poverty. His father was a gambler and an alcoholic who left California in a hurry because of his many gambling debts. For a while they farmed in South Dakota, but the farm failed, and my grandfather left his wife and children to struggle on their own. They settled in Tacoma on a small farm, his famously strong-willed mother raising her four children on her own. Times of deprivation left their mark on my father. He used money to control the people he loved, and emotions were kept deep inside.

My parents, one from the city and one from the country, did not share any of the same leisure interests except playing Bridge and drinking. I remember them laughing together while having cocktails at parties, smiling and appearing happy. But by the end of the night the laughter and the feigned companionship were over.

* * *

I never questioned my parents' unhappiness in their married life. In our family we did not discuss unpleasantness. And we did not challenge the actions of adults. It was easy for me to stay apart and independent, which became a lifelong habit. Much of my young life centered on siblings, school, and friends. Because the neighborhood was safe, I was free to play as a child. There were plenty of girlfriends and boyfriends. At school I was encouraged to sing and play the guitar and sometimes I was featured in music events. I did well in school and lived up to the standards set by my parents. On the outside, everything looked good.

In our home, the three oldest kids were Cherie, Bob, and Kris. They were generally put in the category of "the big kids." Dan was the middle child. Then Mary, Matt (my twin,) and I were the young children. My big sister Cherie was a socialite who did well in school. Bob was the over-achiever; my father viewed him as special, the oldest boy, his namesake. Kris was not as academically inclined as Cherie and Bob, but she was well-liked by her peers and became class president in high school. She broke our family expectation of enrolling in college immediately following high school and instead left home for a life in Europe.

Dan was the overlooked middle child who gained attention by his wit. He was funny and loving but frustrated by his lack of status in the group. Mary was fifteen months older than me. As a young child my mother called Mary "Sunshine," but she permanently lost that endearment in her pre-teen years. She became a wild child, experimenting with sex, drinking, and drugs.

Matt was my twin; we had a special bond. He was big and I was little, yet I protected him when needed. As a young boy he was awkward and uncoordinated. He grew up to be tall, blond, a champion swimmer, and handsome. Then, for a while, he became my defender.

I was seldom in trouble as a child. From observing and learning from my older siblings, I knew which childhood risks I was willing to take and how to avoid being caught when necessary. I always thought of myself as able to reject temptations, yet I do recall wanting to experience alcohol at a young age.

* * *

By age eleven I began experimenting with drinking and smoking cigarettes; both later became my addictions. I tried marijuana in my early teens, but I did not like the feeling of introversion it created in me. Alcohol opened me up. I was thirteen when I experimented with an illicit drug. It was a pill and that's all I knew. A close childhood girlfriend said she tried it and found it fun. We were going to a party that night at another friend's home and I agreed to join in the experience. At the party I felt myself reeling out of control and acting strangely. My friend was hallucinating. My twin brother Matt was also at the party and he was frightened for me. He later begged me not to do something that stupid again. I agreed and have never again used any other substances besides alcohol and tobacco.

By high school, I was busy and not interested in getting high. The high school drug culture of the middle-class life in the 1970s held no allure for me. I focused on grades. I worked as a waitress and I bought a horse.

Owning a horse was no small accomplishment for a city girl in Detroit in the 1970s. My father was against it. He was unwilling to help me financially with her upkeep. I believe this was a reflection of his younger struggling years. He had a pony and other animals growing up on the farm but viewed the expense of a horse as foolish for a city girl. Money was the priority for him, meant only to be spent to obtain useful and productive goals. Nevertheless, my beautiful mare, Jes, was my pride and joy.

While my friends were partying on the weekends, I was waiting on tables, working at the barn, or riding Jes. I was learning to take care of myself. Since personal problems weren't discussed in my home, I didn't turn to my parents, especially my father, for advice. My mother was available for simple dilemmas, but not for those deeply intimate. I was always concerned that my thoughts or actions would disappoint my parents, so I shared little. My parents lacked intimacy and trust, their patterns were anger and judgement. It was easier to remain under their radar, so I did as I pleased within boundaries.

In my father's eyes, buying my horse was a first act of defiance. That act was followed by another when I bought an old, beater car at age sixteen. We had another car, a new one, which Mary, Matt, and I were expected to share. However, I wanted my independence. My old Pinto wasn't pretty and probably not as safe as the family car, but I didn't care. Rather than being proud of my independence and accomplishment my father felt his control over me diminishing.

My father learned to establish power and control over his wife and children through the distribution of money and possessions. I defied his control by going outside that pattern. He did not force me to sell my car, but I was not allowed to park it in the driveway. I believe the reason was two-fold. First, my father worked as an attorney for Chrysler and my car was not a Chrysler product. Second, I had not asked for or received his permission to buy a car. So, this was my punishment. Luckily for me, our next-door neighbor was an elderly lady who didn't drive, and she allowed me to use her driveway.

By the time I was sixteen I owned a horse, a car, and bought my own clothing. I asked my parents for little by choice. By this time the big kids and Dan had grown older, left home, and virtually all communication had vanished within my parent's marriage. My mother talked openly of divorce, especially when she was depressed. It was a time of emotional distance in our home, I stayed apart from both my parents. They were preoccupied with surviving a broken marriage in what was soon to be a childless home when Matt and I finished high school. We never discussed what I planned to do after graduation.

*　　*　　*

Some of my fondest childhood memories were at our cottage on Duck Lake near Traverse City. We spent summers there, swam, played cards as a family, and ran through the woods. We stayed with my mother at the cottage while my dad worked in Detroit and drove up on weekends.

Ours was part of a small community of lake cottages. Most nights for this group of cottages we called "The Colony," there was a happy hour for the adults at 5 p.m. All the neighbors from lake cabins took turns hosting.

Life was grand on summer evenings as the adults celebrated with alcohol. Little did I know how this model for social celebration was to become a part of my life.

* * *

I felt lost after high school. I'd established some independence by buying a horse and a car of my own. I was not to be controlled, I was proud of my accomplishments and wanted more.

But besides being independent I had no clear picture for my future. All my friends enrolled in college with their family's support. Despite achieving almost all A's in high school, I now had no future plans. With the emotional drama in our home it was easy to escape the serious conversations about my life. No one was having those discussions around our home.

For years I'd watched the game my siblings played, one of submission to blackmail, pretending emotional connection long enough to get the promise of a monetary support from my father for college. But I threw down the glove, showing the world I was too strong-willed to plead for money. My father remained silent. I wasn't willing to do go through what I viewed as groveling for college. I succumbed to a powerful family pattern while believing I was choosing to live life my way.

Perhaps Ancestry.com will one day map family behavior patterns as part of a person's lineage. For me it was a pattern of independence, a need for personal control, and difficulty being vulnerable in social relationships. Without understanding I was living within this pattern or realizing the burden of this pattern, my decisions to go my own way were part of a multi-generational response to fear and hurt. I'd learned to use the quick retort, the use of words and emotions to be in control of situations and to choose emotional isolation over vulnerability. Instead of recognizing this family pattern, I absolutely believed I was setting my own course as I began to live as an adult.

So instead of going to college I moved to Traverse City. It was close to my parents' cottage with its peaceful memories of summer life on the lake. Deciding I preferred rural life to urban streets, I found boarding for my horse in Interlochen and worked two jobs waitressing. I went to Europe for a month to visit my sister Kris in Spain and returned in the winter planning to work and enroll in the local college.

As I settled into my own life in Traverse City, my mother finally filed for divorce. She followed me north and for a few weeks stayed with me in my small rented house. She viewed me as her confidante, which quickly became burdensome.

Instead of the life of independence and emotional distance from family drama, the drama managed to follow me. Mom and Dad tried to use their children as allies in the emotional war they'd declared or as objects of their hostility. They used me as an intermediary.

My mother used me as a sounding board and confidante. I received angry drunk calls from my father at all times of the night. I could never fully satisfy them. I felt again like the child trapped at the dinner table enduring my parent's ugly relationship though I had tried to create a life of my own. I was going to college, working, and partying on the weekends. With my new friends I went out to drink and dance and have fun, but also to escape the hurtful behaviors I wanted to leave behind.

* * *

I was out dancing at the Fireplace Inn when I met my husband-to-be. My life was busy with college, working, and playing whenever there was time. He was a country boy, recently discharged from the Army. Kind and generous, but also a bit wild, he seemed not a bit concerned with success or money. He was a country hick, as I had been taught to think. His ambitions were questionable, and I had goals. He was not college educated. In every way he was so different from my father and the standards my father wanted for his children. I quickly fell for him.

My relationship with Brent was complicated by his clearly stated desire to stay unattached and play the field. At times he made me very happy and others he crushed my heart. But I was smitten. Somehow, I believed that my expectations should become reality. Before long, I moved in with him and found myself pregnant. I believed we would grow up and become responsible parents. I believed he would forego his excessive drinking for marriage and fatherhood, but that never happened.

We married against my parent's wishes when I was twenty-one. Defying my parents' expectations, I married a roofer, a non-professional, and I was pregnant. I dropped out of college and was again working as a waitress. My parents viewed my marriage as a disappointment, a topic too uncomfortable to discuss directly with me though it was an endless source of criticism and judgement within family discussions.

My father gave us money for our wedding, but as always, the money was given void of pleasure. My mother accompanied me to a seamstress and altered her wedding gown for me. I was beginning to show my pregnancy by the time of the wedding and the fitting of the gown was filled with overtones of shame and disappointment. I'd chosen my own path. I was independent and beyond their control. I was also pregnant, uneducated, and broke. We didn't talk about it.

My marriage to Brent lasted nineteen years during which we had our daughter and two sons. We built a successful roofing business and had a comfortable life. Many years were happy but being the wife of an alcoholic often left me emotionally lonely. As was my pattern, I did not speak of my deep unhappiness until the marriage was beyond saving.

With my parents I shared only successes because I feared their criticism and judgment of failures. I felt a close bond with my older sisters as the youngest. But in our family, most relationships were built on the family architecture of substance abuse, secrecy, pretense, and fear of rejection. Later, I came to fully understand the conditional nature of my relationships with my sisters at a time when I needed them the most.

Most of my siblings were heavy drinkers but managed to live high-functioning lives. My oldest sister had a master's degree in nursing. Another became a college instructor. My brother Dan started and ran a successful business. The exceptions to our family's alcohol abuse were my non-drinking oldest brother, Bob, and my twin, Matt.

Bob was ten years older and somehow recognized how alcohol controlled the family. He disliked the sarcastic and hurtful words that always materialized after hours of drinking along with the irresponsible and self-centered behaviors. We thought our raucous family gatherings were bonding moments; Bob viewed them as mean-spirited. Our uncensored drunken comments could be hurtful and inflict pain. They were also a way to release it. During these family gatherings, we laughed at pain and discomfort rather than address it. I have since learned that these are typical patterns of alcoholic families.

Later, while I was locked in prison, Bob was the only family member to visit me regularly. He was the only sibling to ask if I needed anything. He offered to help my children. He became the person I told about my fears, pain, and insecurities. I could not yet see it, but his strength and unconditional love would give me much needed courage in the years ahead.

*   *   *

Two tragedies occurred when I was twenty-seven and again when I was forty-one. Both deepened my sense of isolation. First, I lost my twin brother to a drowning accident. Matt was a champion high school swimmer and enjoyed outdoor challenges. He had come to Interlochen for Thanksgiving. On a beautiful, sunny Thanksgiving morning, Matt woke early and went to the family cabin on the lake for a canoe ride. The cottages along the lake were filled with people during the summer months but were cold and empty by the end of autumn. No one knew where he was, and he never returned. Five miles away, large with the pregnancy of my second child, I was busy at home with my family and extended family up for the holidays. Thanksgiving festivities were planned for later that day at my mother's house.

I took a bath to relax after starting the day. I'd been thinking of Matt continuously, looking forward to seeing him and imagining the comforting back rub he would most likely give me. As my twin, we had an inseparable bond. We'd continued our closeness after leaving home. Matt had big, gentle hands that could rub the knots out of my back. It was like I could almost feel his comforting hands while lying in the bath water.

I believe it was during that time Matt was drowning. His canoed flipped and doctors later said he died in the frigid water within two minutes. Sometimes I still feel his presence in quiet moments of thoughtfulness.

My brother Dan committed suicide at the age of fifty. He was successful in business and much-loved by the people in his life. Dan had a special way of making others feel good about themselves. He'd built a prosperous business in Texas in spite of his alcohol habits. For Dan, there were always new ideas and plans for the future. When the economy tanked in the early 2000s his business collapsed. The pain of failed responsibility fueled his drinking. Few understood the crushing weight of responsibility he felt. As he saw it, I later learned, he had failed his family, his parents, and his employees. We all believed Dan was resilient. He seemed invulnerable to me, but that is how people seem when vulnerability is much to be avoided.

My belief that my brother would recover from this setback was never questioned until he died. His alcoholism took control. Help was available, but Dan struggled to accept it. All this was occurring as I began my own spiral downward in my alcoholic journey. Our family, with its secrets and denial, masked normalcy as we buried our brother. We did not talk about our own challenges with alcohol or the possibility of tragedies to come.

* * *

I loved my oldest brother Bob, but in most ways, I never truly knew him while I was growing up. Bob was out of the family home when I was eight. Later, he was the only white sheep in our family living a healthy lifestyle. Like most of the family at the time, I looked forward to the entertainment and fun of drunken assemblies. Bob rejected it. But this was how we knew to be close as a family. As the liquor flowed, the laughter increased, and problems disappeared.

Some of us drank liquor, some wine, and others beer. Many in the family could mix their drinks. I stuck with vodka and orange juice as I never liked the taste of alcohol, only the euphoria. The orange juice disguised the flavor. Every celebration, commiseration, holiday, and birthday involved drinking. It took a substance for us to enjoy ourselves or cope with sadness. We held on to these behaviors because we knew nothing different. We considered those who didn't drink to be stuffy and boring.

As an adult, most of my friendships revolved around drinking. My life was busy with family and business, yet something was lacking. I seldom felt particularly close to anyone. In my personal narrative at that time, I'd accepted a life where the needs of others were my priority, my children and my husband. But, in reality I was a product of old familial patterns.

When it came to getting support from others, I didn't know how to ask or where to turn. Holding onto a mask of control, I avoided conveying any feelings that showed vulnerability. As the years passed, I became lonely and unhappy, mirroring the life of my mother. Brent was a faithful husband and a hard worker. I knew he loved me, but deep down I felt alcohol was his priority rather than me.

When I met Steve, we were drawn to each other. We were both lonely in our marriages. We developed a friendship that grew into a love affair. It was ours alone, our secret. We spoke of our feelings and longings in a way I had not shared with a man. We felt the wonderment of a new love and found happiness in each other's arms. Our marriages soon ended in divorce.

My second marriage had highs and lows. Steve's grown girls blamed me for the demise of their parents' marriage. My boys, now in their early teens, felt a loyalty to their father and the absence of him. They rebelled against me as I spent much of my time focusing on my new husband and our future.

Steve and I quickly took on several real estate projects and started building a new home. We worked hard, and we played hard. We spent much of our free time at a local Eagle's Club.

Steve involved the boys in hunting and snowmobiling, activities they had seldom known with their father, but our new family was having trouble blending. There were fewer family dinners, less communication, and their mother was drinking more, which meant drinking all the time.

Sara, my oldest, was also losing her way. She was my staunch supporter and I had disappointed her. She needed guidance as she graduated from high school. I was too wrapped up in my new life to recognize her needs. My narrative shifted from selfless mother to finally focusing on my own needs. Like each person's narrative, this was looking at the world from my own perspective. And my own perspective was also seen through the lens at the bottom of a vodka bottle.

My family was falling apart, and I struggled to maintain my denial of this obvious truth. I blamed the struggles of uniting two families. I blamed Steve's failure to recognize the effect these challenges were having on me. I blamed myself. Feeling the growing distance between myself and my own children might have motivated me to find help, to reach out to healthy friends and relatives, or to find a professional with the experience to guide me through these difficult waters. Asking for help was not my pattern.

I was failing my children and failing my new marriage. I could not find balance in my new life. Stress began to outweigh my contentment. I needed alcohol to calm me and my drinking quickly escalated to a new level. I feared the extent of my drinking being found out.

*   *   *

Fear was part of every day in Level Four. I was living with women who had committed horrific acts including the killing of strangers, loved ones, or even their own children. At any moment a prisoner might spontaneously attack or assault with planned intent. Level Four made me aware of a depravity within society and people that I had never comprehended.

I had a choice. I could try to hide in the confines of my cell twenty-four hours a day or keep company with the forty or so inmates in Level Four. Rather than isolating myself, I went outside to the prison yard whenever possible. It was hard, pushing myself along with my walker, walking slow miles on the track in the yard, and often conversing with women I would not have known in my other life in a small community in northern Michigan.

Many of the women described broken relationships. They spoke of parents who were not present emotionally or physically. They described fathers who were unknown or had abandoned them. Mothers who were struggling with physical, emotional, and economic survival. Friendships that were transitory, unreliable, and based on shared addictions. Some of these patterns were familiar and I could relate to their stories. But many of the women also described childhoods in which learning was not a priority, growing up with families with illiterate parents and siblings, and growing up with little sense of opportunity for a good life. I met women who lived only to survive, hoping to find thrills on the streets of their poor neighborhoods. They once dreamed of finding moments of peace in the arms of a man or through the rush of drugs and alcohol.

These women taught me about the laws of the street. Survival was a priority by any means possible. Making a living was often only available by becoming a dancer, selling drugs, or stealing. Staying safe often meant hurting others before they could hurt you. Children were valued, but they could also be a burden for those with little family or community support. They described struggling to maintain a roof over their head, to keep food in the refrigerator, and to maintain a basic sense of safety. Their struggles were beyond my imagination.

In Level Four, I also met a few women whose backgrounds were similar to mine. Though most chose not to share specifics of their crimes, it was never long before some of the details were revealed. It was difficult to discuss life before prison without divulging some particulars. It was also impossible to live in such a closely confined community without learning from the prison gossip grapevine. For those who were looking for dirt on another prisoner, a simple call home could initiate research on the details of an inmate's incarceration.

There were few secrets among the women of Level Four. I began to realize common traits I shared with them; we didn't know how to ask for help and we lacked steadfast support systems. We may have lived in different neighborhoods, with different schools and different clothes, but the patterns that led us here overlapped. In one form or another, we experienced a lack of trust and connection. We feared rejection and showing vulnerability. We saw our options as limited. Powerlessness abounded often stemming from addiction. Fear replaced logic. In Level Four, these patterns had led to a world of bad choices and heartache.

* * *

I began to play cards with these women who had sold their bodies, sold drugs, and in some cases, participated in killing another human being. We gathered to play at the tables outside our cells under the watchful eyes of the guards. There were limits on how many inmates could gather at a time. Too many inmates in one place was considered a danger. Two officers were stationed in our unit per shift. They sat behind a desk on the middle floor with unobstructed views of the upper and lower levels. The officers could observe our cells and the gathering spaces, but not the interior of the bathrooms.

Our common areas included the tables space and two glassed-in rooms. One was for television and the other for hair styling. I never knew the TV to work in the television room and the hair styling room was most often occupied by women who were either braiding or using hot irons to straighten each other's hair. These activities were allowed during the few hours a day we were not restricted to our cells.

Playing cards in prison reminded me of the card playing I had known with my family. It was competitive and cut-throat. We frequently played spades or euchre, but I also learned pinochle. As a young child I learned bridge, which involves counting cards, so my skills of recalling which cards had been played were better than most. Around the card table in prison I began to learn, as I like to describe it, to grow a set of balls. While we played only for fun, I bluntly called out others for cheating.

There was always low-level mischief among the inmates, including cigarette smoking in the cells and bathrooms or tattoos being applied with sewing needles and gel-pen ink. Sex took place in the bathrooms or in the cells and occasionally in the open when officers were thought to be distracted. Guards were unable to punish inmates for a new hickey or a fresh tattoo unless caught in the act. But sometimes there was an urgent whisper or the tone of a voice that predicted something more serious was about to happen.

Not being part of the inside cliques, I was never privy to any of the significant plans being devised to break the rules. I existed outside the underworld of selling commissary and drugs, or the world of homosexuality, or revenge. But not being involved did not mean that I could not be affected by trouble.

One afternoon, while in the bathroom alone, I heard screaming and yelling outside in the hallway. The shrieks were chilling and close. A large woman, a lifer named Lee, chased another woman into the bathroom. Lee was holding a combination lock in a sock, a common prison weapon, and swinging it ferociously trying to injure the other woman. Looking for an escape, I realized the exit was blocked by the women. Luckily, Lee accidentally dropped her weapon and while trying to retrieve it, I fled with my walker to the safety of my cell.

Frustrated that she no longer held the lock, she tackled the other women and bit her, inflicting a potentially deadly curse. Lee was HIV positive. Later I learned the fight began with a simple disagreement of words. Lee sought revenge and things escalated into the attack.

Everyone knew Shirley ran a store out of her cell, including the officers. She kept more commissary than any one prisoner could possibly consume. But she carefully procured the necessary receipts proving each item was legally bought.

A couple of prisoners devised a scheme to steal Shirley's key to her cell and use it to steal her commissary. Cell doors in prison are locked to keep unauthorized people from entering more than to lock someone in. Every prisoner was issued a key and directed not to lose it. A key safely in your control was the only insurance that your property was safe. If a prisoner did misplace a key, she lived at the mercy of the guards to lock and unlock her cell until another key could be issued. This could take days or weeks.

The women planning to steal from Shirley waited patiently until she left her key unprotected in a common area. They quickly stole it, holding on to it for days. The loss of the key was reported, but because there was no apparent, immediate threat Shirley immediately let down her guard and left her cell unprotected and exposed. The women entered Shirley's cell while other prisoners stood lookout for the guards. Breaking the lock on her footlocker, they stole all her commissary. The bounty of cigarettes, food, and personal hygiene products was quickly dispersed throughout the unit so it would not be discovered all in one place.

When Shirley became aware of the break-in, she became violent; screaming and yelling. The guards immediately put all inmates on lockdown and conducted a cell-by-cell search. I knew nothing about the plan or who was involved, but my bunkie, Alice, did. Her comments made me guess some of the stolen merchandise was hidden in our cell. She told me no names or details, and I was happy not knowing.

After days of investigation, two women were taken to segregation. One was a lifer, known to be trouble. The other was a woman just beginning an eight-year sentence on a theft-related charge.

Though the perpetrators had gone to segregation, the situation was far from over. The several inmates who aided in the plot were still in Level Four. They began seeking revenge on those who had reported the perpetrators. I'd been implicated. Someone claimed I sent a letter to the warden describing the details of the break-in. I soon learned from another prisoner that a hit had been arranged on me. I did not know at the time a prisoner being released from solitary agreed to hurt me.

* * *

Rumors circulated about a prisoner being released from Level Five after ten years of solitary confinement. She was a lifer, a murderer. While in prison, she'd assaulted both prisoners and officers. Dark, as she was called, cared nothing for prison consequences. She was dangerous and unpredictable.

Even in Level Four, Dark's arrival to our unit created a wave of trepidation. I stayed far away when she was placed in our unit, but I was fascinated, and I observed her from afar. She'd been in solitary for a long time and seemed uncomfortable in crowds. Her reputation shielded her; both inmates and the guards treated her cautiously, unsure of her state of mind. They wanted to minimize trouble and stay on her good side. Dark isolated herself in her cell for long hours. Her bunkie, a woman I knew, lived in fear every hour they spent together in the cell, unsure how to predict her behavior.

Dark was a thin, very black-skinned woman about thirty years old. She was usually silent, paying attention to others but showing little expression. She rocked her body back and forth continuously while sitting. I wondered if her rocking was a habit from her long years in solitary confinement and if it calmed her. When she was among others, she sat quietly, seldom speaking. Mostly she kept to herself. I never saw her smile.

How our association began still confuses me. Dark represented danger to me. But one day she walked straight up to me and asked me to talk. She spoke in a low voice about the previous night when I was playing cards and she was sitting close by. We needed a fourth chair at our card table, but no one was willing to ask Dark to give up one of the two that were stacked underneath her. I finally addressed her, looking directly into her expressionless eyes. I asked if we could have one of the chairs. She gave it to me.

Dark said she had been observing me. She watched me helping Gail, another black woman, struggling to prepare for her General Equivalency Diploma, or high school GED. I often helped Gail in the unit at night with her studies.

Gail had a quick temper. She was slow to learn and easily frustrated by the cruelty of others. Family, friends, and a husband had lived off her monthly disability checks while treating her horribly. She'd been emotionally and physically abused all her life. I liked helping Gail. It was a long time since I felt nurturing, a long time since I had anything to offer another person. Her face lit up with pleasure when she could successfully learn her multiplication tables or read with understanding.

She'd told me of her crime. Gail had attempted to kill her husband after years of physical and mental abuse. She needed the fear and pain to end, she knew of no other way. Gail had described how her husband used her money to buy his booze. He'd drink himself into a rage and then he beat her. For years she endured this life of bruises, broken bones, terror, and agony. When she shot him the first bullet wasn't fatal, then the gun misfired when she attempted to shoot him a second time. Gail did not comprehend how lucky she was. If she'd successfully killed him it would have meant life in prison for her. Instead, Gail received a twelve-year sentence for attempted murder.

Gail was a victim in my view. Poverty, mental disability, and unending abuse sent her over the edge. In our unit, several women liked to taunt her knowing she would react spontaneously without thinking about the consequences. When I tutored her, though she was limited, she learned. The simplest success brought her great joy. I enjoyed her company and successes.

Dark warned me that I needed to watch my back, that I was in danger. She told me that she'd made an agreement to hurt me before leaving Level Five. She spoke of the letter I was accused of writing to the warden and asked me if I sent a letter. I told her no, that I knew better than to involve myself in such a situation. Dark understood I had nothing to gain and everything to lose by taking such action. She said she appreciated I had been real with her the night before about needing a chair, as few people were genuine with her. We spoke for a while and she told me she liked me, and she would watch my back.

My life, my experiences, my vision of the world had not prepared me to live with the fear that I felt in Level Four. I knew I was lucky to have Dark's alliance. I expected I needed it. I considered the different ways someone might try to hurt me. Would it be a lock in a sock or a prison shank meant to cut me? Nobody was going to warn me of an attack, but Dark had. Even though I understood her to be mentally unstable, I found great comfort in her willingness to offer me protection.

When I first heard that I'd been named as someone who might have sent a letter to the warden about the theft of Shirley's commissary, I was afraid, but somehow failed to really understand how at risk for peril I was. Being attacked in prison was something from a bad movie, another world. Now I got it. Dark's words made it real.

There was no bullshit in her warning to me. I began to realize no one was safe in prison and that included me. For years I'd lived in fear of being discovered as an alcoholic, in fear of being seen for what I'd become, in fear of losing the love of my children, in fear of the loneliness that consumed me. Now it was a different type of fear.

Survival comes first in prison. Most of the women around me understood this better than I did. They'd been surviving for years. The absence of safety, trust, and caring relationships created a different standard for behavior—the law of the streets.

The most dangerous woman I'd ever met had just explained to me that my life was in danger, that people wanted to hurt me, and that I was not safe. She wasn't kidding. I wanted to believe that Dark's protection would keep me safe, but the intensity and honesty of her words helped me understand I needed to be alert to everything and everyone around me. No longer did I have alcohol to numb my fears or give me courage. To survive the next seven years, I had to find a new way of caring for myself.

CHAPTER SEVEN

"I doubt God, myself and the world I once trusted. Many inmates appear to accept their circumstances, but I don't. My shame is overwhelming while others speak of none. There is a void in me, a hole."

– Patty Steele, Journal Entry, September 2008.

I never became accustomed to strip-searches. It was demeaning and humiliating each and every time. A strip-search required being fully naked in front of a female officer of unknown sexual orientation. While unclothed, I had to open my mouth and stick out my tongue so an officer could inspect for contraband. Next, I had to face away from the officer, bend at the knees and spread my buttocks while coughing so that anything hidden in my rectum would be released. Lastly, I faced forward and spread my labia. It was required each time an inmate had a visitor to prevent and catch the passage of contraband.

Since arriving in Level Four, I finally began to receive letters. A few family members and friends reached out to me, but the messages were painful to read and brought tears. Of course, I knew I should write back, but I had no desire to communicate with anyone except my children.

What could I say? No one could possibly understand

how I felt. I didn't want to write about the past and I envisioned no future. It shamed me to describe the life I succumbed to due to my own recklessness. My need for connection was opposed by my shame and the fear that no one really cared. In prison, I was barely learning to survive and the thought of exchanging pleasantries about trips and restaurants did not fit my daily reality.

Mostly I chose not to respond. A few persistent souls continued to write. Phillip, a friend from AA days, kept me posted on his life and the news in Traverse City. Polly, a long-time friend of my mother's, who had known me since I was a baby, wrote to me from California. Bob sent words of encouragement, pictures of his family, money, and books. He seemed to understand he had to be patient with me. And my daughter Sara wrote consistently, sending cards and photos to remind me of the good days.

My visitor list was finally approved three months after my arrival in prison. The process included submitting a limited list of persons along with addresses and phone numbers for authorization. Each potential visitor had to submit to a criminal background check. No one with a felony charge could visit unless they were immediate family. Finally, in September, my short list of family and friends were permitted to come see me. Yet the only people I truly wanted to see and be with were my children. My shame kept me from wanting to face the others.

Certain days and times were designated for Level Four visitations. Inmates excitedly anticipated spending time with family and friends. The women prepared by spending hours primping and ironing clothes. A hug and a kiss were only allowed upon arrival and leaving. I'd found the lack of physical contact in prison to be unnerving. The gentle touch of kindness was gone from my life.

"Steele, you have a visit." The first time I heard that over the loudspeaker my initial reaction was to avoid responding. The other prisoners often spoke of seeing their people, eating treats from vending machines, and taking pictures for mementos. I didn't care. I didn't want anyone to see me in my prison uniform, with my walker and my limp, and talk about my life in prison or the ugly story that brought me to this place.

But I couldn't hide. Someone was here to see me, and I did not have a clue as to who. Saying I was out shopping was no longer an excuse for not being home. I changed into my blue prison dress clothes with the orange-striped identification of an inmate and reported to the officer's desk. The officer gave me a pass. Leaving the unit and walking to the visitor room, I wished I didn't have to go.

Before allowing me to enter, a guard outside the visitor's room shook me down, patting my body, arms and legs.

* * *

The visitor's room seemed threatening and humiliating. There were numerous metal-framed chairs all facing in a direction that could be easily observed by the officer on duty. It was already evening and only a few visitors remained. Visiting hours ended at 8 p.m. There was less than an hour before the visitors would be told to leave. Prison vending machines lined up against one wall of the visiting room. It seemed a long time since I had seen ice cream, chips, and such a variety of candies.

I was horribly nervous waiting for my unidentified visitor. My mind drifted to thoughts of being behind multiple locked doors, behind fences of concertina and barbed wire, with multiple checkpoints and many guards. Looking around I was reminded I was a convicted criminal and one so hideously bad that I merited being locked away like this. By now I should have learned how to live with such discomfort. I'd already withstood being charged, tried, convicted in court before many observers and further exposed through multiple news reports that made me sound like an unremorseful drunk. But being visited in prison was one more layer of humiliation, one that was justified by the harm I'd caused.

I took a seat and waited. In a few minutes Betty Jean entered the room. She was my late father's girlfriend. She'd been his frequent companion in the last twenty plus years of his life. Betty Jean brought company and joy to his life for which I was very grateful. B.J. walked over to me and hugged me. Tears instantly began to flow, and I sobbed throughout the visit. The fact that someone had to visit me in this institution was crushing, yet I was glad to not feel forgotten. I tried to control the convulsive weeping with little success. Betty Jean pretended I was fine. She talked for both of us through most of the visit. Soon, visiting hours were over and she went home. I was drained and ready to return to the refuge of my cell. But after having a visitor it was time to endure the required strip-search.

* * *

While Betty Jean returned to her world, I walked back to my prison cell. On the way, my crying once again became uncontrollable. It was nighttime and dark, so I hoped no one would notice. But a female sergeant heard me and approached me. She asked what was wrong. I shared only that I had just been on a visit. She began reassuring me that the visitor would return, I would see my visitor another time. I didn't tell her that it was not the leaving of the visitor that was affecting me, but that I hoped no one besides my children would ever come visit me in this hellhole again.

My brother Bob was my next visitor; he came soon after Betty Jean. During his visit I cried softly most of the time. I did not speak of the distress I was feeling; I could not tell him how seeing him made my anguish feel raw.

Bob told me he had driven north to visit my kids. He'd talked with Robert, my youngest, and took Sara to dinner. I greatly appreciated his efforts to check on them. We chatted about his family. I couldn't talk about myself or prison, and thankfully he didn't push me. Bob brought books he hoped to give to me, only to learn the prison wouldn't allow it. He said he would order me books and send them directly from Amazon, which was permissible.

In order to see me, Bob endured the process of entering the locked doors and gates of prison for the first time. After going through the sign-in and check ID process, he waited a long time before being called to the visitor room. The prison system serves its own needs and does not offer basic civility toward visitors or anyone else. Sometimes it took half an hour to notify a prisoner that there was a visitor, and sometimes it took an hour and a half. If a visitor unknowingly showed up during prisoner count, he or she might wait for hours until count was complete before beginning the visitation process to enter.

Bob had to pass through a security point, go through a metal detector, and be patted down. He was told to take off his shoes and socks, empty his pockets and open his mouth for inspection. The guards were taciturn and rude. He had no idea of the extent of the rigid rules, the pain and fear, which were now part of my life in prison. At the time I could not begin to tell him the details of this life.

Though this visit was extremely emotional for me, I also recognized that visiting his little sister in prison was devastating for Bob. The unpleasant process of coming to visit a prisoner was just a prelude to the sadness of seeing me in pain, shamed by my actions, and living with fear in an environment I could not begin to describe. We hugged before he left. It felt wonderful to feel his arms around me. For a moment, I felt safe. Bob is a big man, but he hugged me with the tenderness of a brother who wanted to protect his little sister and with the sadness of knowing he had no choice but to leave me behind. Before leaving, Bob promised he would be back soon.

* * *

My guilt for the shame I'd brought upon my family peaked whenever I thought of my mother. I was the child who had lived close to her. I was her baby girl. In my own way of thinking, I was the daughter she could depend upon. But instead of taking care of her in her old age, I had become a drunk. I had killed a man and badly injured his wife. I was now locked up in prison for a very long time. When my sister, Mary, and my mother showed up for a surprise visit I was emotionally unprepared.

My mother visited me only once during the month I was in jail awaiting sentencing even though she lived nearby. She and my sister were there for my sentencing, but I felt at the time their motives were more curiosity than support. They offered no words of comfort. Neither came to the hospital to visit me after the accident.

They offered no assistance to me or my children during the five months leading up to my trial. Shortly after the accident I reached out to two of my sisters for financial help and was refused. During the difficult days around the death of my father, after my arrest but before my trial, I felt their judgement and resentment for the shame I'd brought the family, but very little emotional support.

Frail and weak, my mother was eighty-six years old and unlikely to see me again as a free woman. She'd traveled four hours from her home in northern Michigan to see me. It was undeniable the toll it took on her to come to the prison, to visit me in this foreign and frightening environment and yet she made the effort. Her eyes were swollen with tears though she tried to smile when she saw me. Her worry for my safety was evident by the way she looked at me and frequently glanced around the room. She feared I was being mistreated. It was beyond strange for her to be in a room with leering guards dressed in black and gray uniforms, or to sit among prisoners who were deemed socially dangerous and unfit for society. For so many years I had wanted to be a good daughter to her, to please her, and now I knew my mother might die one day without me by her side.

My sister traveled with my mother to see me and for this I was grateful. But I'd felt abandoned and rejected by her when I needed her most. I recalled the days when we were close, and I could depend on her. Those days were clearly over. She also had alcohol issues and her rehabs had failed, as had mine. We avoided talking about how alcohol affected our lives. A wall was erected between us and we were unable to have an honest conversation. I felt forsaken by my sisters. Mary and I barely talked in the visitors' room. And then they were gone, and it was time to again succumb to the required strip-search before returning to my unit.

* * *

Finally, at the end of September, a much-anticipated visit was set with two of my three children, Sara and Robert. I was beyond excited to see them, to hug them, to touch them. They had been through so much with me and I missed them terribly every day.

Sara and Robert arrived around 2 p.m. after their four hour drive from home. They could stay only a couple hours before returning north. Entering the prison was a shock for them, but they took it in stride. They mentioned nothing of the rows of high fences and barbed wire or the pervasive sense of doom upon entering the grounds. We talked mostly of home. Robert and Sara were living in my house, the house they'd grown up in. They were attempting to be responsible young adults, but I knew they felt a burden. Though my house had no mortgage, they had the responsibility of monthly expenses and daily upkeep. Robert was left in charge of handling the bills. He was only nineteen years old.

It was troublesome for me to hear of their struggles with money and jobs. Guilt weighed on me once again. Not only did they have to live with the shame of their mother being in prison, but the additional burden of caring for my affairs was placed upon them including a civil suit. I should have been caring for them rather than the other way around.

Both were working. Robert managed a local restaurant; Sara's job was in-home health care. Robert was hoping to go to college. They were finding it difficult to get along in the same house. All I could do was continue to ask for their help and hope they understood I needed it. Too soon, it was time for them to leave. Winter was coming, the roads would be bad, and I knew it might be months before I might see them again.

I called my oldest son, Brent Jr., immediately upon returning to my unit. He distanced himself from me due to my drinking and we hadn't talked in many weeks. I missed him but he didn't answer my call.

*   *   *

During my struggles with alcoholism and my early years in prison I began to feel that I had been forgotten by God. I was raised Catholic and been taught to believe in a forgiving God. But I'd neglected my family, hurt people in my life, become an addict, and killed a man through my choices. The pain, loneliness, and fear I'd experienced for so long now were my punishment. I deserved it. I prayed to God for forgiveness, but I felt none. In my journal I wrote of the desire to feel God in my life, but all I felt was a void.

While in Level Four I was able to attend a Catholic or Protestant service once a week on Sundays. For a few months every Sunday morning I went to a small classroom in the Education Building. A priest and about ten inmates from Level Four gathered for mass. We sat together and prayed. Then throughout the week I witnessed these same prisoners commit horribly cruel and unkind behaviors toward others. I stopped attending and never again joined a prison religious service.

My mother sent me a prayer written out on cardboard a couple weeks before she passed. She was prepared to die, though I do not believe at the time she knew her death to be imminent. During our phone calls she told me she was tired and that I needed to get home soon. We both knew that wasn't going to happen, but we avoided speaking the truth.

She'd tried to send me a plaque with this prayer inscribed on it, but the prison rules restricted me from having it. For years this plaque hung in her kitchen. It read: "God help me to remember that nothing will happen today that You and I can't handle together." On my cardboard copy my mother wrote on the bottom, "I will always love you, Mom. I pray to the Blessed Mother to take care of you each night and the next day."

*　*　*

After seven months of high security, I was moved to a different unit. Level Four was overcrowded and I was deemed less threatening than most of my peers. Level Two offered fewer restrictions and more time out of my cell. I was now eligible for gym activities, some programming, and more time in the Law Library. However, every change brought its challenges. I felt uneasy about the move. I knew this would be an adjustment for me, learning a new environment, having a new bunkie, and adjusting to new officers.

It was a cold, snowy day as I dragged my duffle bag from Level Four to my new unit. A new beginning just a hundred yards away. Auburn B, a Level Two security unit, became my home for the next six months.

An incident took place three days after I left my old unit and shortly before Christmas. The Level Four,

Cord B prisoners were returning from night chow when an inmate named Nimi attacked her girlfriend on the snowy walkway between the prison buildings. Nimi had recently moved from Level Five down to Level Four. These two inmates maintained an on and off relationship. On this night, Nimi carried a blade removed from a razor and a lock in a sock. As they returned from dinner, she jumped her estranged girlfriend on the outdoor walkway and began beating and slashing her with the improvised weapons. The girlfriend was taken to University of Michigan Hospital where she was treated with close to a hundred stitches mainly for cuts on her face, but also her stomach and back.

Nimi was in prison for smothering her three children and there was a general understanding among prisoners that she was a ticking time bomb. Both the Cord B inmates and officers surmised that it was only a matter of time before Nimi would try to hurt someone. She was a dangerous lifer. A few hours after the incident, I spoke with one of the guards who witnessed the attack and was now in our unit.

The young officer, a five-foot-four blond who weighed about one hundred fifteen pounds, was crying. She'd been ordered to videotape the scene after Nimi was restrained. She described the gory scene. She said she was shaking so badly that she could hardly hold the video recorder. While she was telling me of the incident her phone rang, she was ordered to return to Level Four. I heard her tell the person on the phone she couldn't go back. This officer was new, and I wondered if that decision would cost her job.

The bloody snow remained on the walkway for days until rain washed it away. Each time I passed by, it reminded me that I was living in an alternate world from the one I had known. Pain, shame, violence, and fear were the currency of this world. Even outside of Level Four, it was still a world of last visits, of unpredictable attacks, of strip-searches, and endless humiliation.

Hobbling with my walker past the bloody remnants of Nimi's attack, I realized I could end it all, even here in prison. While the guards strip-searched my body and searched my cell, no one ever checked my walker. I could buy medications from prisoners until I had a sufficient supply to kill myself. I could store them in the hollow legs of my walker while waiting for the right time. With a few discreet purchases, my pain, shame, and fear could be over.

CHAPTER EIGHT

"Others tell me I might be here for a reason. Maybe I just don't want to accept this. Maybe I wouldn't be alive if I were home, would that be ok? I would like to be optimistic, but I also like to be real."

– Patty Steele, Journal Entry, December 2009.

Security Level Two brought relief from the limitations of Level Four. The housing units were identical, but the atmosphere was more open, social and flexible. Once the units were unlocked in the morning, they remained that way until 10:50 p.m. except during formal Count Times at 11 a.m. and 4 p.m. These lockdowns lasted about forty-five minutes until the total count of the prison was cleared by the Control Center. This allowed freedom of movement throughout much of the day within the units in Level Two. An informal quick headcount took place at 9 p.m. All activity had to cease for about ten minutes as we stood outside our cell doors while the guards confirmed all inmates were in the housing unit for the night.

The walkway to and from the yard was accessible every hour for fifteen minutes in the afternoons and evenings for Levels One and Two inmates as long as it was not dark outside. This allowed more time to be in the fresh air and away from crowds. This was a great change for me as I needed time to exercise my body and calm my mind.

Prison officials preferred and usually required that inmates hold jobs. A job paying seventy-four cents a day, five days a week was all it took to relieve the state of its duty to provide essentials such as soap, shampoo, deodorant, and toothpaste. It was customary in all areas except highest security for prisoners to hold a paid position unless they were physically limited as specified by Health Care.

Many inmates had jobs outside the unit though the majority remained porters within. For the base minimal pay, porters performed all the duties needed for keeping the common areas of the units clean. More money could be earned working in the kitchen, though few wanted these positions. Not many wanted to scrub pots or cook for the masses. Other positions throughout the prison offered decent prison wages but required skills. Those positions were coveted among the two thousand two hundred women. A written exam was required to become a teacher's aide in the GED program for a high school equivalency. Prisoners were interviewed for essential prerequisites for other jobs such as law clerks or assistants to staff. Some of these jobs paid as much as three to four dollars a day. Having a paycheck at the end of a month totaling sixty dollars or more was only for the few. Because of my leg injury, I was given a no-work reprieve upon entering. That suited me fine since I did not want to be forced to clean toilets or work in the kitchen.

The Level Two facilities included a gym, known as the Fieldhouse, which held activities throughout the day. Some of the favorites were volleyball, roller skating, and working out with weights or in groups with videos. The

THE GIFT OF SECOND CHANCES

Fieldhouse resembled a school gym, a large room with hardwood floors. I disliked spending time there because it was the hangout for girlfriends in same-sex duos, some flaunting their relationships. It disturbed me to watch women involved in gay relationships due to their prison circumstances and not because it was natural for them. I realized that prison can breed unorthodox behavior, and it made me uncomfortable.

Some prisoners were required to go to school and prepare for their GED, while others were placed in job training programs to prepare them for working in the world. The choices for job training offered at Scott's Facility included custodial work and food management. Although I had an associate's degree, I was placed in the GED classroom while the prison acquired my high school transcript.

The classrooms were cramped, equipped for only twelve to fifteen students. The teacher sat at a front desk doing little and relying on his inmate assistants who had scarce interest in helping their fellow prisoners. For two months, I did time in the GED classroom tutoring others and working on an appeal for my conviction. The teacher appreciated my help and supplied me with paper and pencils for personal use. This saved me the expense of buying them off commissary.

The teacher asked me to officially become a tutor in his classroom, but I didn't want to spend five days a week working. I wanted free time for researching and writing my appeal and declined his offer.

*   *   *

Many inmates attended some type of betterment

PATRICIA STEELE

group. What the state offered was limited, but outside sources such as Alcoholics Anonymous and church groups organized a few meetings in the prison facilities that addressed substance abuse and patterns of criminal behavior. Some groups focused on women's issues, including abuse and neglect. There was even a lifer's group. The National Lifer's Association welcomed all inmates no matter their sentence, but they dealt primarily with laws and prison concerns pertaining to inmates without any chance of parole.

I joined the lifer's group and met a female judge at one of the meetings from Wayne County. Judge Mack gave a presentation on battered women, a personal experience in her first marriage. She shared her story and spoke of the absence of Battered Syndrome laws in Michigan. This deficiency limited the use of a battered woman defense, the result being long prison sentences or life for women who fought back against their abuser. After the meeting, I spoke with Judge Mack and shared my legal concerns involving my case. I'd been given the maximum penalty allowed by law which was unusual for a first-time felony. The one witness who might have testified that another car had a crucial role in the accident said she no longer remembered it. Judge Mack told me my argument for appeal held little chance of success unless I could afford an attorney who would take my arguments into the court of public opinion, raising issues in the press of improper and unethical actions on behalf of the prosecutor. She explained that in the typical appeals process, prosecutorial misconduct is seldom confronted, although it is recognized by legal professionals as commonly practiced. In my case, local officials wanted to take a strong public stand against drunk driving, and I was a good example of someone who should not have been behind the wheel of a car.

*   *   *

The mood within Level Two units was not as dreary or disheartening as it had been in Level Four. Time passed more quickly as I was involved in more activities and spent less time locked up. The housing units had working televisions and multiple microwaves. Prisoners could gather for coffee in the morning or make microwave snacks such as popcorn when playing cards. Some inmates bought enough commissary items to forego going to the chow hall and eating the provided prison meals. On birthdays, cakes would emerge from the microwaves baked from Duplex cookies. The cookies reconstituted into cake and the filling into icing. Fat Girl Cookies, chocolate chip cookies filled with microwave peanut butter fudge, were also a favorite when one could afford to buy the ingredients.

It was amazing what women could make in a microwave with commissary items. At times a food ingredient stolen from the chow hall completed the ingredients needed for a dish. Food was stolen from the chow hall regularly. Kitchen workers brought it back to the units to be sold. One of the perks of working in the kitchen was the extra money that could be earned off the stolen meats, spices, or anything else that could be hidden under clothes or stashed outside the chow hall for pickup. Being caught meant your job and a major ticket for theft.

After my move to Level Two, prison officials began cracking down on prisoner kitchen theft to save money. The prison officials began limiting the amount of food bought for inmates. Food began running low at meals. This resulted in women writing grievances for not having the proper food and amounts served to them. The prison blamed the shortage on inmate theft, but most prisoners knew that staff were also helping themselves to the groceries and taking them home. Several times I saw officers taking boxes of food from the chow hall.

Recent budget cuts were instituted, and the kitchen was now operating on a smaller budget. This was accomplished by cutting out many fruits, vegetables, and meats. We were eating more hot dogs, beans, and processed foods. Salt and pepper were eliminated. Carrots and broccoli became the standard vegetables. The carrots were so large they reminded me of carrots sold for deer food at home. The broccoli was all stems. The budget for feeding Michigan inmates was now less than two dollars a day per prisoner. More women resorted to microwave cooking for variety and taste.

The prison guard's treatment of Level One and Two inmates differed from higher-security Level Four. Not all guards were friendly or fair, but they probably recognized that prisoners with greater freedoms had more ability to retaliate. Level One and Two prisoners had greater access to the Law Library and greater knowledge of official policies and procedures. Most officers understood that the women wished to do their time without issues and avoided overtly abusive behaviors. A few officers demonstrated moments of understanding and treated us as human beings. It was these officers who gained my respect.

*   *   *

My new bunkie in Level Two was called Coins. She was a street hustler who sold both drugs and her body. She was an addict. She'd been to juvenile detention for four years as a young girl and prison for the first time in 2005. This was Coin's second time around at Robert Scott Correctional Facility. She was serving eighteen months for a drug charge and was only in her mid-twenties.

Coins was shot in the face during a prostitution tryst. As a child she had modeled clothing for local advertisers. Now, Coin's face was deformed and covered with scars. She'd endured multiple operations to cover the gaping hole on the right side of her face, but her lost beauty could not be restored. Her face was patched with different shades of brown-colored skin. Her jawbone was deformed, and several teeth were missing. She drooled out of one side of her mouth and black hair grew in odd places.

Her parents were both addicts as well. As a young child, Coins lived with her mother. They were poor and she knew many stepfathers. During a period of her childhood she lived with her grandmother. The years with her grandmother were her happiest memories. Her father did not stick around long after she was born, but she later developed a positive relationship with him. He lived in the neighborhood and fathered at least eight children with other women.

In her early teens, Coins' grandmother died, and she was forced to move back in with her mom. During these years she started getting high with both parents. After a while she turned to the streets to support her addiction, prostituting and dealing drugs.

Although we were from different worlds, my new bunkie and I got along well. We kept each other company in our cell as the holidays drew near. Coins worked in the kitchen and we shared treats she stole from the chow hall. In the kitchen, Coins organized the distribution of food between the kitchen, and the front serving lines during serving hours. Her job required organizational skills, and she was proud of her position.

Coins' mother had been released from prison one year earlier and so far, remained clean. Her mother hoped not to return to prison. One of her brothers was an inmate, but she didn't say why. While she was in county jail her father sent her a small amount of money for the commissary, but she had not heard from him since she had been transferred to state prison.

In our cell, especially in the evenings, we spoke openly of our personal addiction histories. Coins spoke of the many times she'd promised to get clean, but she always failed and disappointed the people in her life. She said they were tired of believing in her. She missed being pretty and knew there were more operations to endure. She said losing her beauty was hard to accept, but she was glad to be alive. I questioned my own desire to live and wondered what drove her desire to go on.

I spent most of the days before Christmas in our cell. The sadly decorated Christmas tree in the unit made me lonely for home and for the holidays I once knew. Once when we were a family, our tradition included a Christmas dinner of honey ham, green beans, and home-made mashed potatoes along with all the fixings and pie. Remembering the music, the laughter, exchanging presents, and being a family made me extremely lonely. That was all gone now. The sights and sounds of Christmas brought me no joy. I found I couldn't watch television. The tender Christmas programs made me want to cry and I wanted no one to know how I felt. Nor did I want to explain the happiness I once felt at Christmas with people who had not known such experiences.

On Christmas Eve, I called my mother, but she didn't answer. I felt relieved since speaking to her magnified my shame. I heard her distress and desperation whenever we did speak. She begged me to call more often but I couldn't. I couldn't see through my own troubled feelings to give her what she needed from me. It is said that alcoholism is a disease of the body, mind, and soul. In prison, I was no longer able to consume alcohol, but my mind was still scrambled and confused, and my soul was utterly broken.

I slept late Christmas morning and woke up in a deep depression. At noon the prison served a special Christmas meal of ham, a small baked potato, broccoli stems, and a sliver of pecan pie accompanied by a very small dab of ice cream. The ham tasted like salt, but the baked potato was a treat. I enjoyed the couple bites of ice cream and took my pecan pie back to my cell. The pie and three cigarettes were my Christmas gift to Coins. She was pleased and surprised, and gave me an uncharacteristic hug.

It was Christmas day and the phone lines were extremely long with inmates waiting to talk with loved ones. I used this as an excuse for not phoning home. Last Christmas I'd been in a hospital bed, recovering from my injuries. My children and two nieces spent part of the day with me. No one spoke of the future. No one spoke of the accident. We all silently feared the events to come. My father was sick, but we didn't yet know he was dying. I recalled how my situation weighed heavily on his heart.

On the Christmas before my accident, I'd spent the entire day alone, drowning myself in my sorrows. My kids stayed away, expecting me to be drinking. My husband had divorced me. I didn't know where to turn for a glimmer of hope and I felt dreadfully alone. My mother went to my sister's house for the holidays, though I probably would not have spent time with her anyway. No one called me; I called no one. There was nothing to celebrate, no tree or decorations, only a desire to die.

Before the bad years, I had memories of filling the house with lights and food. Looking forward to the season, I loved being with family and friends. Christmas brought us all together. Christmas Eve included mass and giving thanks. And there was always alcohol. Beer, wine, and vodka and orange juice were an important part of the menu for as long as I could remember.

On this Christmas in prison, I sat in my cell while Coins drifted in and out to visit her buddies. I was surprised in the afternoon to be called for a visitor. Bob left his family to travel to this gloomy place. He endured waiting as long as the guards required in the waiting room, endured passing through the metal detector and the pat-down to see me. I felt guilty that he was here, but it was wonderful to see him. His face filled with loving kindness when he saw me. He took me in his arms and held me tight. For a while that day I wasn't alone. He had not forgotten me or left me behind.

Bob asked me that day how I thought prison would affect me in the long run. I told him I would never again be the same person. I was losing the last bits of the gentle soul I'd once been. I didn't tell him I feared being no longer able to shoulder the darkness.

Later I wrote in my journal, "How do I explain that I

have witnessed evil and it wasn't in a movie or a chapter in a book? I have been stripped of my dignity. I have brought disgrace upon myself and my family. I don't know why this is my life and I long for answers. There is such sadness here, a person would have to live this experience to understand it."

CHAPTER NINE

"I need to stop beating myself up if I want healing to take place. I need to acknowledge that I am and will always be an alcoholic. I have to find the courage to accept myself and my past. It seems as though to heal means to be vulnerable. I am afraid."

– Patty Steele, Journal Entry, May 2010.

The New Year began with chaos. The Michigan prison system eliminated cigarette smoking in February, which led to high levels of anxiety for many of the inmates. Women were stealing tobacco from each other as the prison gradually reduced the amount of tobacco that inmates could purchase. This led to fights and distrust. I was a smoker and from the time I entered prison I began buying tobacco and papers for rolling because a pack of cigarettes cost too much on my prison allowance. I'd asked my children to send fifty dollars a month for my commissary expense. Fifty dollars barely provided me with enough money to buy personal hygiene, a few snacks, and tobacco. Smoking rolled cigarettes with no filter was common in prison. We all had yellow fingers from the tar, and many had chronic coughs. The state, in its desire to decrease health care costs, had decided to eliminate cigarette smoking.

At the same time, Scott's Facility had begun shifting women out of Level Five at an unprecedented rate. Lower level inmates were being transferred to the Women's Huron Valley Correctional Facility in Ypsilanti. There was a sense of uncertainty in the air, of instability, that was creating increased stress levels for prisoners and staff. In the early spring, we learned that the state planned to close the Scott's Facility. All female prisoners in Michigan were to be housed together in one location, at the Women's Huron Valley in Ypsilanti, Michigan, about thirty miles from Scott's Facility.

Preparation for the move began with weekly practice pack-ups. Inmates were expected to pack everything we owned in our state-issued gear, which meant one duffle bag for most of us. We were instructed to place our packed belongings outside our cells for inspection. Cells were then inspected for hidden property.

For me, packing everything into one duffel bag was no problem. The only property I accumulated beyond that issued to me was a sweat shirt and a tiny, state-approved television. It all fit in my duffle bag along with my limited hygiene products and commissary. Some of the lifers and long-term inmates invested one hundred dollars for a state-approved foot locker. These eased the process of routine pack-ups and allowed for more personal possessions.

Many inmates were forced to throw out excess prison clothing they accumulated as well as other personal belongings. Some women had multiple sets of sweat shirts and sweat pants for wearing in the yard or in the unit to stay warm. Some had two or three visiting outfits. Others owned radios or MP3 players as well as their small televisions. Hobby craft items were common. Women bought them for making cards or to crochet and knit.

Many women had extra commissary and these pack-ups were stressful.

The practice pack-ups were then adjusted so that prisoners moved their gear to the central base of each unit. Prisoners were forced to drag their packed belongings up or down stairs to the base where officers inspected every single article. It was common for women to trade in clothing and other items without the knowledge of staff. All property by policy had to be documented with the original receipt. All clothing purchased through the prison system contained a label with the prisoner's identification number. Televisions and electronics sold to prisoners had clear exterior casings to ensure no contraband was inside. Visible engraving of a prisoner's number had to be present. Inmates had ways to get around identification problems on possessions, but not on this short notice. Mounds of confiscated property were collected for disposal after each practice pack-up.

The actual move to our new facility began in May. Unmarked buses were brought into the prison to carry us to our new home. Prisoners were strip-searched before being placed in restraints for the bus ride. We all wore our prison blues, which identified us by new and clear white prison identification numbers on the back of our shirts. The buses were equipped with cages for high-security prisoners or problem travelers. Many of the women enjoyed the bus ride despite the circumstances. They had not seen the world for many years other than from the yard at Scott's. Seeing buildings, new cars, and traveling down the freeway was an adventure for them. I found no joy in the move. I felt like an animal being transported from one zoo to another.

As much as my life at Scott's was filled with discomfort, misery, and despair, I feared the unknown. Many of the officers from Scott's were among the staff, but there were new people in roles of authority at the Ypsilanti Facility. Although the plumbing was lousy and many of the buildings were crumbling, I knew what to expect at Scott's. I was accustomed to the daily routine. And I feared the unfamiliar.

Upon arrival, my new home was less than inviting. It had multiple high fences equipped with electric volts, barbed wire, and gray cinder block, cold and uninviting. We were funneled into the fieldhouse. The process of entering the prison was organized like a human assembly line. We were told to retrieve our belongings and report to an open station where once again every item was inspected by an officer. Each prisoner was assigned a unit and a cell. This prison had two separate sections. The East Side was originally built for women, while the West Side, the older side, had recently housed high security Level Four male prisoners. I was assigned to the West Side where the men had just evacuated.

Walking to my new living quarters, I noticed the prison grounds were greener than at the Scott's Facility. The yard on the West Side was large. The buildings appeared in better repair, and geese were nesting everywhere along the walkways and in the nearby fields. I passed housing Unit Four and Unit Three as I walked toward Unit Two. They all looked the same from the outside, large brown brick buildings facing a central walkway. In addition to these housing units, the West Side included a building which housed the Law Library and another that was the Control Center.

My new residence was two stories high. When I entered, I was immediately struck by the atmosphere.

Inside it was dark and dreary. The building held more cells and fewer gathering spaces than the housing units at Scott's. Each housing unit contained two wings and each wing had three shower stalls. This building, which once housed one hundred men in single cells, would now house twice as many women, and for one hundred women in each wing there were only three shower stalls. This was an obvious problem.

Climbing the long stairway to my new housing unit was challenging. There were no elevators for me, or helpers assigned to the infirmed or older inmates. Dragging my belongings and holding onto the railing in case my leg gave out, I could smell the decades of male prisoners who recently lived here. On the second level there was a catwalk running along two rows of cells. It looked down upon the main floor. A waist-high cast iron railing kept people from falling into the open space between the rows of cells and gave officers a view of both levels.

I was instantly sickened entering my cell. My gaze went first to the bunk bed on the opposite wall. The lower bed, my bed, had four-point restraint mounts used for shackling the previous tenants to the frame. I saw filth everywhere. Dirt and grime from previous tenants remained. A gelatinous slime combined in a putrid jambalaya was visible around the bed and in the corners of the cell.

A small window with bars offered a restricted view of the side of the unit next door. The door contained a rectangular opening for food trays to be passed through to the prisoners. From outside the cell, the pass-through could be accessed to give food to prisoners restricted to their cell. The cell door locked from the outside. Unlike at Scott's, only the officers had keys. Once a door was locked it had to be re-opened by an officer. To my disgust, the cell had a metal toilet and sink. I was to share this space that was essentially an open bathroom with my bunkie.

The only good thing about this day was that I was transported in one of the earlier buses. I entered my new unit before most of the others arrived. The officers in the unit sat behind a central desk as we walked through the door. There was no greeting, no one spoke to us. I found the cleaning supply closet and began scrubbing the cell from ceiling to floor with powdered bleach and water. Bleach was not usually an allowable cleaning agent, since harm could be wrought upon others with it. But I found a stash. Someone left a limited supply and I knew it would go fast.

My bunkie arrived, a young black woman who'd been assigned to my cell at Scott's shortly before the move. She was a lifer, in prison for killing her young daughter. She was a small woman in her early thirties. Cleaning and personal hygiene were not high on her list of priorities. There was a disconnect from reality about her. She came in and sat on her bunk, watching me. When I asked her if she wanted to help, she refused by simply shaking her head. She was however willing to go up and down stairs to fetch clean water and supplies for me. She knew from our short time bunking together I was not eager to live in a cell covered in someone else's dirt. I would do all the work, but the stairs were my obstacle.

Every surface had to be washed. There were writings on the walls, pictures, and crude marks. Black mold and feces needed to be scrubbed from the walls, beds, and mattresses. As I cleaned, more women arrived to find that supplies had been used up. They were aggravated and disgusted. Tension quickly grew within the overpopulated housing unit. The officers solved the problem by locking us down, confining everyone in their cells no matter the physical condition. For the rest of the day, they let us out only to go to chow. The women screamed at the guards from their cells but were ignored. No one was happy, including the officers.

As inmates we bore the repercussions of disgruntled officers. Their hell was our hell. On this day and for many more to come, there was plenty of frustration and aggravation to go around. This facility was to be my home for the next six years.

* * *

During the first month of my imprisonment, officials assessed my substance abuse and the circumstances leading to incarceration. Their one recommendation for my entire seven years was to attend Alcoholics Anonymous. At some point in my incarceration I was to attend meetings for a minimum of twelve weeks. Following this, I would receive a certificate of completion, which might someday help me appease the parole board.

Soon after moving to Level Two and while still at Scott's, I signed up for AA to complete this twelve-week obligation. I was placed on a call-out to attend Wednesday night meetings. As I had little interest in going, I figured to get it over and done with.

This was not my first experience with Alcoholics Anonymous. I went to AA meetings before while in rehab and found them to be comforting. Near my home I attended meetings for a while but felt out of place. Walking into an AA meeting alone I'd felt exposed, defenseless. I hoped no one knew me, might acknowledge me, or expect me to speak. I was afraid of being honest about my continuing desire to drink. I did not want to hear what I perceived to be the sanctimonious stories of others. Several times I attended a meeting after drinking a few cocktails, anxious for the time to pass so I could leave and stop pretending. It was torture, listening to others speaking of their accomplishments, their serenity, and feeling none myself.

I arrived at my first prison AA meeting expecting to feel the same as in the past. It was held in a classroom in the education building during the evening. I knew no one, but that didn't matter. I figured everyone was in the same mindset as I. Few women in prison sought to address personal issues, including substance abuse. Most of the women I talked with believed their use of drugs or alcohol was normal and part of their life circumstance. I figured I was sober. I had not had a drink for over a year, nor had I searched out any of the prison hooch.

Hooch, homemade liquor, was available and made from stolen fruit from the chow hall and yeast. Though I hadn't consumed alcohol in a long time, I was not yet thinking of my long-term recovery. What might happen when I got home felt like a lifetime away. I couldn't begin to think that far ahead.

Chairs were placed in a circle. The meeting began as all AA meetings do with readings followed by sharing within the group. I sat quietly, not saying a word. I wondered if there would be silence or if others might speak. The AA volunteers encouraged participation, but they did not push. There were usually about twenty inmates with few contributing to the discussion. Some of the women sat near acquaintances sharing personal conversations. Some were there to meet up with girlfriends.

The two volunteers who came to facilitate my first meeting were both regulars with long term recovery from substances. They initiated the dialogue following the readings and inspired others to speak. They shared bits of their personal experiences with substance abuse and recovery and spoke of how their use could have landed them in prison. They spoke to us as equals describing the lives they once lived and the happiness they now felt in recovery. Neither escaped dire consequences in their lives, but managed to get through those tough times without coming to prison.

Both volunteers were a bit older than me. They exuded the grace of age and wisdom of experience. One woman, June, was a petite blond. She was used to taking charge and directing the meetings. The other, Nancy, had red hair and a bright twinkle in her eyes. She was warm and grandmotherly. Both had kind smiles. They spoke to us not as prisoners, but as people deserving of dignity. Within the walls of this prison, being treated with dignity was a welcome reprieve. They laughed about their past outrageous drinking behaviors and commiserated with us about the consequences. We all knew our substance use had once given us enjoyment and freed us from ourselves. And we all knew that for us, drinking had severe life consequences and penalties.

After the meeting, June and Nancy welcomed me. They encouraged me to come again, they hoped next time by choice. These women appeared normal to me and they believed in the process of healing from the depths of addiction. I was drawn to them though I didn't understand why at the time. I could sense their integrity. I felt no judgement from them for wearing a prison uniform. It did not seem phony when they seemed to recognize there was a broken but good person still inside me.

For a long time, I didn't speak up in the AA meetings.

The other inmates who attended the meetings only knew my first name and the fact that I still attended meetings even after receiving my twelve-meeting certificate. From this, I expected they surmised I was looking for answers and healing. It was more than a year before I shared anything of true significance. Slowly I began opening up about my fears, my sense of failure, my guilt and my loneliness. I grew to understand the volunteers once felt as I did now and had for so many years. Somehow, they overcame the sunless days and the even darker nights. I asked for their help.

* * *

During the days at Scott's I sought out opportunities to walk outside whenever it was possible. There was a well-worn route around the edges of the exercise yard. Some of the time it was just me trudging slowly around the yard pushing my walker. Other times an acquaintance would join me. But mostly I used this time to be alone with my thoughts. It had been a long time since I'd had a drink and I no longer craved one. Sometimes during my walks my mind seemed to clear, and my thoughts became less frantic.

* * *

I began to look forward to seeing the AA volunteers and they became my support system. They came from different backgrounds and socio-economic status, yet each one walked the path of addiction and was trying to navigate the ongoing path of recovery. I quickly understood they truly cared about me and my sobriety. They focused on similarities, not differences. One woman, Erin, dressed in flashy jewelry, heels, makeup and hair. She reminded me of a Barbie doll. Another woman, Cindy, came after work always looking professional. She was an inspiration, beautiful and eloquent in her appearance and message. Cindy spoke honestly of the challenges of achieving recovery and of the rewards. I wanted what she had. I wanted to be a confident and yet a real woman. I wanted to be a woman worthy of respect. Dawn brought laughter; she lived life with gusto. She came once a month and whispered to me throughout the meeting all the things we would do together when I left prison. Dawn had property not far from my home in Interlochen where she visited regularly. I believed her. We made plans to continue our alliance beyond my incarceration.

These women offered me life-changing lessons, the first being forgiveness, and most importantly, forgiveness for myself. In the meetings, we studied together the twelve steps of Alcoholics Anonymous. They focus on personal accountability and responsibility. They remind us we are not alone in our battle for sobriety. The principles of AA are based upon the belief that alcoholism is a disease which affects the whole of us; our minds, bodies, and souls. They stress we must give up the illusion that we are in control of our lives to regain it.

For me, this meant recognizing I could not surmount my alcoholism on my own. It meant I had to have faith in others and in my Higher Power to guide me. Instead of pushing people out of my life due to my shame, I must tear down the walls I erected. I must share my pain to regain connection with myself and others. I must trust that the people still left in my life would not desert me and instead support me through my difficult process.

When I first attended AA meetings in prison, I expected that this experience would be like all others I knew in my desire to remain sober. The words would be comforting, the camaraderie might be pleasant, but the lasting effect limited.

But these women made me question my deep skepticism about recovery. They convincingly spoke about alcoholism as a disease. I knew a little about the science behind the addiction, but I judged myself as an alcoholic, synonymous with being morally bankrupt. These women reminded me of the goodness within me. They repeatedly pointed out my destructive actions were driven by my disease, not my character. They told me when I could lay aside some of my overwhelming shame and guilt, there was room in my heart for healing.

These volunteers traveled without pay or thanks to be with us in prison. In each meeting they emphasized the need to admit my wrongs to myself, to God, and to the people in my life. I resisted their message. It was difficult to face myself honestly, to become vulnerable and accountable for my behaviors and choices. My fear that I was not able to change my addictive behavior was still too strong. It was more comfortable to deny and avoid the truth. I feared that in facing the reality of my choices, I would lose the people I loved. I somehow ignored the fact that I already pushed away so many people in my life with denial.

* * *

At Women's Huron Valley, my walks kept me in contact with the seasons. Even when the weather was cold, or wet, I walked. My leg continued to ache. Walking made it hurt more for the first few minutes and then the pain lessened, becoming more manageable. Occasionally due to the weather the yard was closed. Sometimes long chow lines limited yard time. On those days I could not walk, my discomfort grew worse and it was much harder to sleep at night.

*   *   *

My daughter Sara was my lifeline to the world I'd left behind. Every few months, she came to see me. We planned her trips during our phone calls, which gave me great pleasure. She shared her life with me, the good while trying to protect me from the bad. In spite of the embarrassment I'd caused her, she could also remember the good times. She missed those good times.

With Robert, my youngest son, communication was more difficult. He remained living in my home and visited about twice a year with Sara. I'd left Robert with the task of running a home for the first time and handling my finances which began with a grim civil lawsuit. The family of Mr. Jones sued me. For the first time in my life I couldn't oversee my own affairs. I sensed my son felt overwhelmed and unappreciated. I worried. Resentments were building.

Brent Jr., my middle child and oldest son, kept a distance I was not able to cross. We spoke infrequently on the phone and he did not visit. It hurt me not to see him, I knew I'd caused my children enough pain and did not know any way to undo that from my prison cell. I wondered if I would ever find a way to reestablish our connection.

* * *

There were a few amazing people who gave me their strength when I could not find my own. Polly was an old family friend, a little bit younger than my parents. She knew me from the time I was a young child when on summer vacations near my parents' cottage in Interlochen. She understood some of the alcoholic dynamics of my family, but even more she knew I needed a friend and a strong support system. And she reached out to me in prison.

Polly asked that I write to her rather than call to communicate. She knew it helped me immensely to put my thoughts on paper. She was a psychologist living in California, still practicing in her 70s. She shared with me her enduring belief in the possibilities for change. Polly always responded quickly to my letters offering insights for me to ponder and grow from.

During each yearly summer visit to Michigan she came twice to visit me in Ypsilanti. She walked into the visitors' room with such excitement, as though I were the most important person in her world. On one of Polly's visits, she told me I was the daughter she never had. I did nothing to deserve the affection of this remarkable woman.

My brother Bob never stopped coming to visit me, month after month. My other family members sent an occasional letter or note saying they were thinking of me, but never asked what they could do for me or my children. Their words felt empty to me. I often wondered how much my relatives were embarrassed by my circumstances. Did they explain to their families and friends that their sister was in a prison for the death of a man because she was an alcoholic and drove drunk? Or had they stopped talking about me altogether, stopped thinking about me?

Unlike the rest of our siblings, Bob never was a drinker. It was plain to see that it was difficult for Bob to enter the prison grounds and then leave me behind in this awful place. His visits validated for me that I was important to him and not forgotten. As the oldest brother, I believed at first that he felt responsible to care for me, but I soon realized his actions went far beyond responsibility. Bob never gave up on me. We spoke about our family, the love and the dysfunction. We grew to trust and depend upon each other with a new appreciation. Bob is ten years older than I am, and in my childhood memories he was often gone to college and then went on to his own life. Bob opted out of the drunken poker nights and other alcohol-dependent festivities with our family. Somehow, he'd traveled a different path. I felt much less alone as our ties grew stronger. But I worried I could not live up to the dreams he had for me.

I reconnected with my first husband after a year and a half of silence. He was with me and our children during the trial. Then, when I entered prison, I did not call him, and he did not reach out to me. Brent Sr. remained important to me though we were divorced. And I held a special place in his heart as the mother of his children.

Our communication began with a phone call I made to Sara. It was a couple days before Brent Sr.'s birthday and my kids were all at his house celebrating with him. I talked to each one and then with Brent Sr. I loved hearing his voice and felt like I had just reconnected with the most loyal friend I had ever known. Because I hadn't expected to speak with him, I wasn't prepared and felt very emotional. I had to cut the call short as I was crying.

Only a month later my mother died, October 22, 2010. A deputy came to my unit and told me to call my daughter, but she would not tell me why. She took me to her office where she tried three times to place the call for me. With each unsuccessful attempt my worry grew. Finally, I begged her to tell me what was so wrong and why she came looking for me. The deputy explained that she learned from Sara my mother had passed that day. I felt a mixture of strong emotions. I was deeply saddened that my mother was gone, but even more I was relieved that nothing horrible had happened to one of my kids.

I had expected my mother would die while I was in prison. She was eighty-seven years old and struggled with emphysema for years. For me, the death of my mother was another tragedy to endure alone. The funeral took place two hundred fifty miles away and I was not there with my family. I wasn't able to be at her side in the hospital. I wasn't able to share in the grief process. I let her down.

I began calling Brent Sr. once a week just to talk. I often shared with him my concerns about our kids. Our phone calls were casual and easy, and I looked forward to talking with him. I was aware it was unfair to create some unrealistic relationship, but we could co-parent and be friends. Many women in prison form relationships with men through the mail, on the phone, or in the visiting room that are fabrications of what they are missing. They want to believe they are special to someone in a romantic way, but these relationships have no lasting foundations. I did not want to pretend with Brent Sr. I had hurt him severely during our marriage when I had an affair and later divorced him to marry my new love. I did not want to hurt him again.

* * *

Shortly after my mother died, Brent Sr. was diagnosed with cancer. He was afraid, and I was afraid for all of us. He was never an assertive parent, but in my absence, he was the person my kids could count on. As a veteran, he was treated at the VA hospital in Saginaw and then in Detroit. His treatment required he go to the VA in Detroit every three months. Those trips always included a stop to see me in Ypsilanti.

Our kids had endured so much in a short period of time. My arrest and incarceration were followed first by their grandfather's passing and then their grandmother's. Brent Jr. didn't want to see me. Sara and Robert were struggling to live peaceably together in my house. During a phone call with Sara, she broke down and wept telling me she wasn't sure how much more she could take. Sara never cried, but the struggle was crushing her. I'd failed them all and wondered how much more my family could endure.

From my prison cell, I had no capacity to help any of them. I could not even help myself. Every day I craved peace of mind, but I could find none. The squirrel cage in my head kept going around and around. The worries, the helplessness, and the hopelessness. I wanted to trust in a God of possibilities, but I was afraid of disappointment. I longed to feel connected, but that feeling remained elusive.

It had been more than two years since I had a drink. The alcohol was out of my body, but the effects were still present in my mind. The squirrel cage mindset of addiction remained.

At the AA meetings I was usually quiet, afraid of letting anyone too close, afraid of exposing myself to their scrutiny, afraid of giving up control, afraid of failure. The twelve steps program seemed insurmountable. I could get to step one, admitting that my life was unmanageable and that I was powerless over alcohol, but the rest was still a journey beyond my reach.

And so, I walked. In the changeable weather of southeast Michigan, with my walker or my cane to support me, in the prison yard surrounded by armed guards and concertina wire, I walked one step at a time.

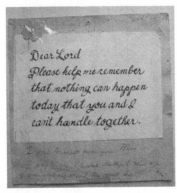

Patty's prison identification card.

MICHIGAN DEPARTMENT OF CORRECTIONS

Grand Traverse
County
PAROLE

NUMBER
686898

Patricia Ann Steele

A note from Patty's mother sent to her in prison.

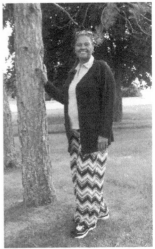

Terri Jones, Patty's substance abuse counselor while in the Residential Substance Abuse Treatment program.

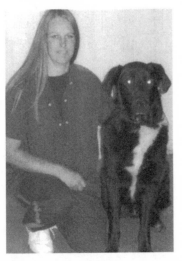

Stiltz and Magoo during MI Paws training program.

April 21, 2012

Dear Sara, Brent, and Robert,

This letter, I expect, is going to be difficult for me to write but I feel a need to express my thoughts to you all concerning some delicate subjects for me.

I had a conversation with Robert not too long ago where he verbalized to me some of his feelings. He told me something I found hurtful and yet, I appreciated his honesty. Robert said, he would never allow me close enough to him to where I could hurt him like I did in the past. I have to say, I fully understand the distrust, but I do want all of you to forgive me completely and understand that my intentions have never been to cause harm or sadness to any of you. I am sorry for the pain and shame I caused you in the past and still do today.

Before the accident for a long period of time, I felt like life was completely out of control for me. I felt as though I couldn't make anyone happy no matter how hard I tried. I felt alone, hopeless, and helpless. My emotions were those of despair and depression and my behavior reflected them. The more broken I felt, the more I drank to numb my feelings. As everything spiraled out of control and my actions affected those around me, my shame and guilt became unbearable. I thought there was no solution to the hell I was creating for everyone and that is when I saw death as a solution. I figured you all would be better off once you got past my death, life goes on.

Since the accident, my life has taken on another form of hell. There have been many times I have felt alone, abandoned, detached, and frightened. I have had to go through the judicial system unaware of what could happen to me and I live daily in a horrible place surrounded by many horrible people and conditions. I have experienced new forms of fear, humiliation, and mental pain that I didn't even know existed. I have had to live with terrible guilt and shame. I have lost friends and family. I have had to face the fact that my life was not filled with loyal and caring people. I have felt many disappointments and faced many truths. I have felt unloved and undeserving of love. BUT, what keeps me going is this: it is when I talk with one of you and you say I love you at the end of a conversation, when I call and you sound happy to hear from me, when I get a card or a letter that lets me know you remembered me on a birthday or birthday and that I still matter. It is when people like Bob help me in any way they can no matter the inconvenience to them, or others who put money on their phones so I can call any time and those who write and visit me and make me feel worthy. You see, here it is easy to feel unimportant and forgotten.

Now I need to let you know what I need from each of you. I need your forgiveness. I need you to recognize that I never <u>intended</u> to hurt you. I understand I did hurt you, I understand you may still be angry, I understand you may not feel ready to trust me, but I still need your love and support. If I am completely and totally honest with you, I don't know if I completely trust myself when it involves alcohol and depression. I'm still afraid of how they might affect my life in the future. I do know however, I can no longer handle others who are

selfish in the giving of their love and leave when the going gets rough. Those who are afraid of what might be asked of them. I feel like I have lost too much to those type of people, they have hurt me too much and I need to stand up for myself and say, no more. The truth is, bad things happen all the time and there is not always someone or something to blame. I'm not saying my actions did not bring about these circumstances, I'm saying, I didn't ask for the alcoholism, the depression, or the accident to happen.

I believe that one of my biggest flaws, beyond the obvious, is that I never have been able to ask for help or expose my insecurities. I think I needed help and wanted it, but I didn't know how to get beyond my pride and pain to let others know how scared and at a loss I felt. In the Sornson family, the women were expected to be strong, but I needed help. I was so scared of my mistakes and inadequacies and I was fearful of sharing them with anyone else. If I couldn't handle my problems myself, how could anyone else? What would others say about all the mistakes I had made? Not good reasoning, I think I now have to realize and understand that to be vulnerable is o.k. I need to voice my fears. I have to think of this as strength rather than weakness. I need to not shy away from taking care of me.

I also need to let you know I have changed a lot through this process. Robert and Sara remarked to me how I didn't cry when I saw Brent. Although seeing as Brent was absolutely wonderful, I have shed so many tears over the past few years that they no longer come as freely as they used to. I do not feel as though I'm as tender and gentle a person as I used to be. There are many changes in me I don't particularly like, but they are reality.

As well, I would like you to know I think about the day when I will walk out of here. I have to tell you all that although it is still a long way off, it scares me. I feel like I will be fragile out in the world. I am afraid of how others will react to me and receive me. Although I expect that it will be a very happy time, the unknown will be scary. In truth, throughout this experience, it has been the unknown that has been the most frightening. I hope to have your full support. I expect it will be important for a successful transition. You may not realize, but after so much time away, reconnecting to a previous life, including friends, family, work, a home, a position in the community, feels daunting especially when the reason for the absence has been a tragic accident and prison.

Patty's last Christmas letter to friends and family from prison.

December 5, 2014

Dear Family and Friends,

I am grateful to be writing my final Christmas greeting from prison. It has been a long seven years in which I have witnessed and experienced more than I could ever imagine. I have along the way also gained knowledge of myself and of a world I didn't know existed. I hope the "transformed" me is a wiser and better person. I want all of you to know, it has only been with your love and support that I have made it through this difficult time. I don't know what I would have done without you.

I want to take this opportunity to thank everyone who advocated for me with parole letters. The letters were beyond fabulous. I have no doubt the parole board was aware of the wonderful family and friends who support me. Thankfully, as you all know, I have received my official walking papers. I will leave this hell-hole behind me on April 14, 2015!

I would like to include in this letter a special thank you to my brother. Bob went with me to the parole hearing. Bob has encouraged me throughout this process as only an amazing big brother is able. When I first saw Bob's face the morning of the hearing, I knew he was more nervous than I was. Thank you Bob, I could not have asked any more from you. You were a great representative. Your little sister loves you very much.

You will all be in my thoughts and prayers this holiday season. May the holidays bring you every blessing possible. Now, I would like to close this letter with a prayer sent to me by my mother a short time before she died. She sent the prayer on simple gray cardboard, so the prison would not reject it. It has hung on every bulletin board in every cell I have occupied and it used to hang in her kitchen. It reads:

> Dear Lord,
> Please help me remember
> that nothing can happen today
> that you and I
> can't handle together.

God has seen fit to get me through these years, he has given me each and everyone of you and for that I will be eternally grateful.

Love,
        Patty

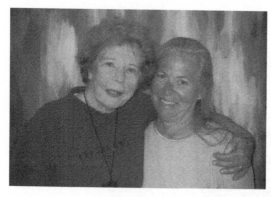

*Patty and her
special friend
Polly during a
prison visit.*

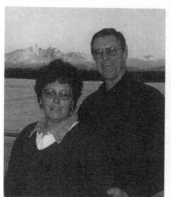

Patty's friends Carol and Gary.

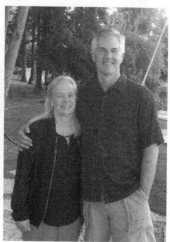

*Patty and her oldest brother, Bob,
at his home.*

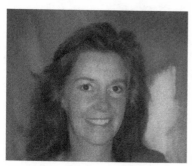

*Stacey, Patty's close friend and
prison bunkie for two years.*

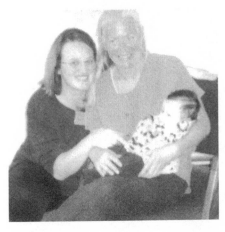

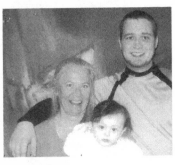

Daughter Sara,
Patty and newborn
granddaughter
Savannah.

Patty, granddaughter
Savannah, six months, and
her youngest son, Robert.

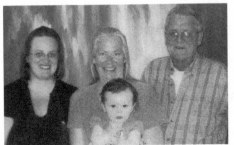

Daughter Sara,
Patty, granddaughter
Savannah, nine
months, Brent Sr.

Patty and granddaughter Savannah eight months before her release.

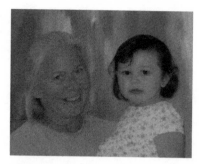

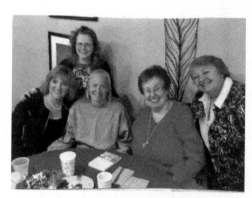

April 14, 2015, Patty's prison release day. She is celebrating with Alcoholics Anonymous volunteers who helped her in prison.

Patty's release date at a restaurant in Ann Arbor. From left, Bob, his wife Nancy, Brent Sr., Patty, Savannah and Sara.

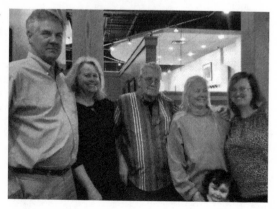

CHAPTER TEN

"Carol brings God into my life in a way He was never there before. She makes me think about my spirituality. She tells me to stop trying to make sense of our circumstances for that is where faith comes into play."

– Patty Steele, Journal Entry, April 2009.

Often, I felt hopeless. For so many years I was the parent who made decisions for my family and now I could only pray my children and ex-husband would make reasonable decisions and find good outcomes. For so many years, though my life was affected by alcohol, I believed it was under control. I believed I could control myself and my children and be the quintessential successful American family.

Here in prison there was no pretense of control. They told us when to get up, when to eat, what to eat, how to dress. Every moment of every day we were reminded that we deserved to be controlled like sub-human creatures. There was no pretense of control here. My family was struggling and though I tried to influence their decisions I knew that my words lacked impact. Sometimes I raged inside, other times I felt remorseful, but mostly I felt irrelevant. Sometimes the pain of my isolation, the pain in my body, and the pain of my lack of ability to help my family kept me up during the entirety of my long awful nights in prison.

After months of arguing with Robert, Sara moved out of my house. He'd taken in roommates to help cover the expenses. I wondered how my home was being cared for and what I might come home to someday in the distant future. We'd made an agreement that Sara would always have a place in my home before I left. Perhaps it was more of a demand on my part, a condition over which I now had no control. I worried about whether the taxes and insurance were being paid. Robert vaguely reassured me leaving me questioning his responses. Again, I had no control. I worried about Brent Sr. His cancer was being treated at the VA, but he avoided giving me the details. He was brewing kombucha at home to supplement his treatment. I didn't even know what that was and had no way to research anything in a prison where we were denied all access to the Internet. Brent Jr. seldom spoke to me on the phone and never came to visit. He was working, living with a girlfriend, and telling me everything was fine. Those were the same non-specific words I used when people used to ask me. I could only wonder what was happening inside of him.

I was disappointed with the lawyer who represented me at my trial. He'd been a judge before going back into private practice and my father had believed he could use his connections and experience to get me the best treatment possible. Instead, I got the maximum sentence for my crime. I was angry at the prosecutor, who saw me only as a drunk driver. His valiant attempts to get another drunk off the roads became my fate. My name and my image were widely used in the local media as the example of irresponsible drunks who should be removed from society. They were right in so many ways, but I'd become a two-dimensional cartoon villain. Nobody cared that there was more to the story.

In an effort to force someone to consider my story, I found a lawyer to represent me and filed an appeal to the Michigan Supreme Court. Another prisoner recommended him, and he specialized in appeals. In prison, there was no way for me to research any attorney more carefully. I paid this lawyer a lot of money upfront after meeting him only one time with the promise of energetic advocacy. There were legal timelines for my appeal, and I wanted to review and control some of the content. I sent him the first appeal I wrote with the legal arguments I expected him to expand upon. I called regularly for updates, but he either did not answer the phone or told me he was still working on it. I asked Bob to step in when he failed to respond to my letters and phone calls. It became clear that he was only going through the motions. No joke intended.

A few years earlier, when the family of Mr. Jones filed a civil lawsuit against me, I had to hire another lawyer and a civil suit consultant in northern Michigan to defend me. There was very little money left, and most of it was taken in the settlement. After that was done, this lawyer also billed me for additional payment. It just went on. From prison I was restricted to waiting for letters and documents to arrive and trying to call or write letters in response. My son, Robert, helped immensely with the civil suit, but after a while he hated it all and resented the position I'd put him in. When resentments built up, I'd ask my brother to get involved to clear issues with

Robert, or Sara, or a lawyer, or Brent Sr. But I hated asking for help. Wanting control of my own life, having so little, dealing with resentment, wishing for healing. All these added to my confusion and to the emotional madness that brewed in my horrible cage of a life. For me the cage was not a metaphor, as I was reminded every morning and every night.

*   *   *

Sometimes I was grateful. When I met Carol Hart, alias Carrie Fox, we were in Level Four. She intrigued me. She was in her early sixties, had a gentle inviting smile, and a small heart-shaped tattoo positioned below the corner of her left eye resembling a tear. Carol accepted her circumstances better than anyone else I had come to know. She had just been recaptured and returned to prison after escaping nearly forty years earlier.

Our friendship began as she joined me for my slow walks while we were still in the Scott Facility. It continued when we moved to Women's Huron Valley. Both of us were housed on the West Side and Carol's cell was near mine in Unit Four.

Carol was the mother of four, a loving daughter, and a dedicated wife. More than anything, Carol was a devoted child of God. Though Carol did not expound on her beliefs overtly, her spirituality was plain in her actions. When I looked at Carol, I saw a woman who could have been my sweet neighbor at home or a person I might meet in church. Nothing about Carol resembled a criminal, much less a fugitive. Carol had a tender demeanor, a quick wit, and a kind and caring attitude toward everyone. Her history fascinated me. I wanted to know everything about her original charge, her escape, her reasons for absconding, and what it was like to live thirty-nine years on the run. Prison etiquette called for us to avoid cross-examining each other about the past.

Finally, after we'd built a friendship, I broke etiquette and questioned Carol about her story. Sometimes she laughed while describing her memories and other times she cried when the past was tough to relive. She tried to forget the bad days and said my inquiries brought a roller coaster of emotions for her. She often had to dig deep inside to recall details. Carol spent thirty-nine years on the run trying to erase her past.

She had shared her history with only a few people over the years. While a fugitive, she decided that the less people knew about her criminal history, the safer they would be from possible consequences stemming from aiding or harboring a fugitive. I found this woman to be a mountain of strength. She said her strength came from her faith in God.

Carol grew up in a rural area on the fringes of Flint, Michigan. Her parents were strict, especially her father. Carol married young, in part to get out of her parents' home. She soon had two children and an abusive husband.

Some of her friends lived on what Carol described as the wild side. Carol socialized with those friends without her husband. Though Carol was not a drinker, she spent time at bars with these friends and was often the designated driver. On the night that changed her life, Carol and friends were at a local bar. After leaving the bar, she planned on driving with one of the guys to another friend's apartment. She knew this man carried a gun. Carol thought him dangerous and he scared her.

When he directed her to stop at a motel along the way, she feared he intended to get a room and force her to have sex with him. But when she stopped near the motel office, Curtis got out and went inside, telling her to wait.

Through a picture window she could see him arguing with the motel owner. Carol became scared and decided to drive away and leave Curtis behind. As she left the property, she heard gunshots. Carol did not stop. She did not go to the police. The next day Carol was arrested.

The police informed her that Curtis attempted to rob the owner and killed him in the struggle. Carol had no money. The court appointed her an attorney who convinced her to take a plea deal. She pled guilty to assault with the intent to rob while armed and received a sentence of twenty-five to thirty-five years. Carol was told she was eligible for parole under good-time behavior in about twelve years.

Before accepting the plea, Carol met with the county prosecutor. He offered her a way out of her circumstances. For fifty thousand dollars he could make her case go away. Carol could not raise that amount, nor could her parents. She'd believed the plea deal was her best option.

While still in the Genesee County Jail awaiting transfer to prison, a major fight took place on the woman's block of the jail. This fight affected Carol for the rest of her life. A female inmate broke a glass bottle and attacked other women in her cell. I saw fear in Carol's eyes as she described that day. It was as if she was reliving the experience again. Carol was slashed on the neck in the chaos although she was not sure if the person who attacked her was the woman with the bottle or another inmate who retrieved a piece of broken glass from the floor. She recovered, but was constantly afraid. It was fear that motivated her plan to escape.

In the early 1970s, prison fences were topped with barbed wire rather than concertina and much shorter than they are now. It took about a year to formulate her plan. Carol escaped through a chow hall window and over the fence.

Carol picked an evening in September of 1970. She dressed in multiple layers of clothing to protect her body from the barbs topping the fence. Two other women followed her that night, but she said she didn't remember their names nor know what eventually happened to them. She recalled that one woman had only a year sentence and she tried to talk her out of running away.

After climbing the fence and running for the cover of nearby woods, the three women spent the night walking and crawling through woods. Several miles from the prison, they found a barn to sleep in. The next morning, they walked down a country road and two young men stopped and picked them up in a pickup truck. The men asked questions about them being dressed similarly and the women made up a story about being sisters.

As she told me this story over several days at times her memory faltered. This was especially true when it came to names of the individuals who helped her. She explained that it was more than forty years ago, and she did not remember some of the details. I believe that Carol was protecting them. She decided she would go to her grave never telling anyone specifics of who then assisted her in buying a bus ticket to Florida and gave her money to start a new life.

Her life as an escapee was difficult. She changed her name to Carrie and spent many years manufacturing a new identity. She was compelled to lie to people she liked and to avoid letting coworkers or neighbors get too close. She was always in fear of the law tracking her down.

In Florida, Carol met a woman who came to her aid. The lady bought Carol a car for three hundred dollars and assisted her in obtaining fake identification. She helped find Carol a job at a local gas station, though it was short-lived. The owner of the gas station wanted Carol to wear skimpy clothes to work; this made her uncomfortable.

Shortly after arriving in Florida, Carol moved in with a man. Their relationship began as roommates, but it soon became sexual. After a few months it ended when the man told her to get out of his house because his wife was returning home. She did not know he was married. Carol confided to me she made many bad decisions in those days involving men. She came to believe she was not worthy of a good one.

Carol went by a new name. She worked in bars and restaurants for a while in Florida, and at one of them she met Chico from Puerto Rico. They bought a home together but were never married. She had two boys with Chico, sons she adored. Carol found it hard to be out of contact with her first two children back in Michigan, but she knew her parents were caring for them. After only a few years of living on the run, when she thought she was safe to contact her family, Carol telephoned her parents and told them she was safe and in Florida. Carol's parents and older children made occasional surreptitious trips to Florida to see her. It was difficult to explain to the kids that they must never speak about her or where she was living.

And there were difficulties in her relationship with Chico. He had a substance abuse problem and disappeared for days at a time. Sometimes he became violent when he was high or drunk. She described to me the last time he beat her. He pounded her head into the floor and left her covered in blood. Later he returned home ready to be forgiven; Carol told him it was the last time he would hurt her. In response, Chico lunged at her, but Carol opened a kitchen drawer and pulled out a knife. Chico backed off.

Ending relationships as a convict on the run can be confounding. Will your former lover rat you out? Or use your circumstances to take away your children or black-mail you?

She found another place to live with her children and worked in a series of clerical positions, including book-keeping at a beauty school. Moving frequently and chang-ing jobs was part of her strategy for avoiding detection. She took a job as a secretary for United Way, her all-time favorite job. About this time her friend died of cancer. Carol took in the friend's teenage daughter to raise. These were challenging years for her.

Once Carol began sharing her story with me, it began to emerge with the power of a chronicle which had been long repressed. Every day we walked and every day we picked up the story. Sometimes I asked questions asking her to dig deeper into memories, but more often I just listened with respect for this woman's strength.

As a single parent with little money she focused on ways to stretch a budget. Carol recycled everything possible so it could be used a second time. She and her children wore second-hand clothing from thrift stores and left-over food was seldom thrown away. She told me of using rags for cleaning instead of paper towels, as paper towels were too costly and extravagant for her. Her frugal habits con-tinued in prison. She counted pennies even though her husband sent her ample money. She bought few extras for herself, yet she was generous to others. Carol regularly supplied her bunkies with toothpaste and shampoo. I teased her about her penny-pinching ways and jokingly told Carol that when I was able to visit her someday at her home, my arms would be full of paper towels. She responded, "Don't bother, I won't use them!" She was obstinate, but as kind and loving as any person I knew.

Carol's most recent home was in Manton, Michigan, a short drive from my home in Interlochen. We often talked about reuniting once we were out of prison. We would walk along the shores of the Manistee River. We dreamed of sharing our lives as close friends and helping each other heal.

After Chico, Carol met a man named Ken. They decided to move to North Carolina and marry. But Ken was a womanizer and the marriage did not last. While Carol was married to Ken, she met another man named Gary to whom she felt a different kind of attraction than she had found with the men in her life. Carol had a job as an in-home health provider for this man Gary's elderly mother.

She shared that Gary never approached her for a date until after she was divorced from Ken. He stood out from the many men she knew and was a humble man with traditional values. He spoke with a thick hillbilly accent, read his Bible daily, and attended church weekly. Gary had no substance issues and believed that marriage was a sacred trust. Carol and Gary dated for five years before she finally accepted his repeated proposal of marriage.

Carol explained to me why she couldn't make a commitment to Gary for a long time. She could not marry this virtuous man without honesty about her past and her concerns for the future. She loved him but decided to remain single to avoid bringing him into the mess she'd made of her life.

He persisted. Finally, she agreed to marry him on one condition. He had to be made aware of the possibility that some day she could be rearrested and why. Carol told Gary about her arrest years earlier and her escape from prison. She spared him many of the details and he asked for none. Gary promised if he were ever questioned by the law, he would respond that he had little knowledge of her past and none of her criminal history. Carol was frightened by the thought of Gary being at risk of being charged with a crime due to his love for her.

* * *

On our walks, Carol and I spoke with complete honesty about events in our lives. These were emotional days for both of us. We let down our guards with each other and found trust rather than shame. We talked of being young, of making mistakes. We talked about our families, how we hurt them, and how they had sometimes hurt us. We shared our fears and dreams. We talked of pain, anger and disappointment; we shared our insecurities. I told her of my dark days, my loneliness, and my struggles with alcohol. She told me of the faith guiding her through the intolerable days, a faith that gave her the ability to endure. She believed that we would have opportunities for happiness in our futures. She told me that God never left me, but my pain blocked my ability to feel his presence.

Carol is the person who showed me how to look beyond the prison fences. When walking outside she gazed up and expressed her gratitude for the beauty of the blue sky or the white puffy clouds. Sighting a rainbow with Carol was joyful even if standing in the pouring rain. Together we talked of home and the natural splendor of northern Michigan. She called it God's world. Those talks brought to mind the luscious greenery and the color of the fall, the rivers and lakes with their inviting waters. Sometimes in the early evenings when the last sun spewed streaks across the sky, Carol looked up and told me they were the staircase to heaven. Still today when I see the last rays of sunlight in the early night, I think of my friend.

A beautiful sunset of reds and oranges were the promise of a new day. Carol became my sister and dearest friend. When she spoke of God, I believed her. Many nights after being with Carol, I prayed for a new relationship with God, one that offered a sense of safety and comfort. Because of Carol, I began to pray again, believing someday there would be an answer.

CHAPTER ELEVEN

"Today Carol and I were walking and talking of home. She is so excited and yet becomes so nervous at the thought of returning to the world. She is concerned about repairing relationships. She is afraid of how her small community will react to her freedom. We shared the fear we hold of others, their opinions of us due to our time in prison and our criminal history."

– Patty Steele, Journal Entry, April 22, 2010.

I spent my first few years in prison acclimating to an environment for which my middle-class background never prepared me. I grew up in an upper-middle-class neighborhood and attended an all-girls Catholic high school. My parents expected me to get a college education, marry a professional man, and live in a gracious suburban neighborhood. I'd blown those expectations to hell, but still had basically lived a safe and secure life. Before prison, I had no need to develop survival skills to protect myself from others. The dangers in my life came mostly from within.

Many of the prison inmates around me spoke of the good times at home and plans for when they got out. I could not relate to those conversations. I was ashamed of my past. My future seemed unpredictable and non-existent. I couldn't visualize a happy future for myself. I could not yet imagine a Patty Steele who was able to create a happy future. I had no idea how to progress beyond Patty, the struggling, depressed alcoholic and now Patty, the prisoner. I didn't know how to remold myself into someone I could love. Not knowing what the future might bring kept me paralyzed in the present.

Most of my energies were focused on getting through each day, surviving the dangers around me, enduring my sorrow and physical discomfort, the tasteless food, the barked orders, the strip-searches, the lockdowns, and the clang of confinement when some faceless guard shut the cell doors at night. For me it was day to day, ashamed of the past and fearful of the future.

Helping others was a way for me to get beyond my own troubles, a way to begin healing. I found many different ways to assist some of the women I met. I listened to their stories, their outpour of defeat and humiliation. I remained quiet and supportive when tears flowed telling of life circumstances I couldn't begin to comprehend. I researched legal issues for people who didn't know how to do it for themselves. I wrote appeals and grievances. I spent hours preparing women for their parole hearings. I encouraged positive, constructive actions along with patience and perseverance. I urged forgiveness of others and self. I found I understood the healing process even if I could not yet put it into practice for myself. While I offered support, I learned difficult life lessons from these women. I became aware how much culture and envi-ronment affects who we ultimately become. I began to understand the injustice of the law. I learned about weakness, including my own, and became less judgmental and critical of others and myself. I recognized that bad things happen to good people. I gathered courage to speak up for myself, to share my opinions and insecurities.

Prison was viewed by most as a temporary existence; we were all just passing through. Few inmates developed long-lasting relationships in prison. This was my reality. It was unlike anything I had known before; it was purgatory, not a place for building trust and relationships. I struggled with living in this provisional world while knowing my old world remained beyond my grasp. I found it problematic to create a new identity for a future in a world from which I felt disconnected.

The insistence of others that I might someday build a life of contentment kept me afloat. But this message was clear from only a few, and I remained confused. Carol saw something in me that I could not yet begin to see. And there was Bob, always there for me. Polly, B.J., and Brent Sr. made great efforts to let me know I was not forgotten. And, perhaps most importantly, Sara's love never left me. They had a vision for me of returning to my home, finding a purpose and rediscovering joy. In my purgatory I plodded along hoping they might be right but surer they were delusional.

So much of prison was just boring. With nothing much to do, inmates spent their days idly playing cards, crocheting, preparing microwave meals and sitting around waiting for endless hours to pass. Stuck in my unhealthy thought patterns, I needed some way to fill my days that would bring positive energy into my life while helping to pass the endless moments.

*   *   *

While helping other inmates with their appeals, grievances, and parole hearings I discovered in the Law Library that it was possible for me to take college classes. I liked the idea of occupying my time while advancing my education, but it would not be simple to achieve. To take classes, I needed to find a university that would accept me with my criminal history and one that also offered courses by mail. Prison rules required that all books and materials be new and received at the prison from approved sources. There would be no computer access available for researching and writing papers, and no direct contact with a professor.

For a university, there were only a few choices. I wrote to all of them requesting information. Adams University in Colorado ultimately fit my needs. Adams offered a program by mail that included a variety of bachelor's degrees. I decided to pursue a Bachelor's in Business Administration. I was well versed in payables, receivables, and payrolls. I'd worked outside the home for six years as a bookkeeper, as well as keeping the books for the roofing business of my first husband. Adams also offered a minor in Legal Studies that would allow me to take courses to become certified as a paralegal. I could go even further and receive an advanced paralegal certification. I liked the idea of gaining this accreditation and someday possibly working as a legal assistant.

Amazingly, I knew of no one else in the prison who was taking advantage of college classes by mail. Once upon a time, prisoners were eligible to receive Pell grants and many inmates used these grants to pursue higher education. Fortunately for me, my father left a large sum of money to help with the education of family members, mostly to be used by his grandchildren. My brother Bob was the fund trustee. He took care of the finances for me. He enrolled me and then arranged for text books and other school materials to be shipped to me.

All the idle hours spent on my bunk could now be used productively. My legal classes were especially interesting, but I found that learning outside the classroom and without access to a computer or the teacher was challenging. It was difficult to discern what material a professor might include on an exam. This was particularly problematic when taking Constitutional Law. I prepared more for exams in prison than I had ever done before. My exams were taken in the Law Library monitored by the librarian.

There were many papers to be written, especially in my legal courses. I learned to prepare wills, trusts, briefs, motions and more. Most papers had to be typewritten for submission, which presented a special problem. There were no computers available for general prisoner use and only a few typewriters in the Law Library for two thousand women and their legal documents. The only solution was to purchase a typewriter. In the digital age it seemed crazy to purchase an archaic device, and prison policy would make it especially complicated. Any typewriter used in the prison was required to have a clear casing and be bought through an approved vendor. The visible interiors were so they could not be used to hide contraband.

And the purchase of a typewriter through the prison system would be ridiculously expensive. I remember explaining to Bob during a visit a typewriter might cost about five hundred dollars. This was because the state assigned me court costs totaling six thousand dollars on top of my sentence. To collect on this debt, the state took half of all money sent to me monthly over fifty dollars—the amount I needed for my basic commissary items. To buy a two hundred fifty dollar typewriter I would require twice that amount because the state would take half. Bob was stunned at my explanation and then we started to laugh at the ludicrous restrictions that prevented inmates like me from pursuing education while behind bars. God knows they wouldn't want prisoners to stumble upon some road to rehabilitation.

*   *   *

Only much later did I understand how much healing occurred for me during my many walks and conversations with Carol. Unlike me, she accepted both her past and her present. Her soul was peaceful in a way that I could only long for in my own life.

After marrying, Carol and Gary returned to northern Michigan to live near Carol's parents. They built a small home down the road from her parents so they could care for them in their aging years. Carol took a job stocking merchandise at a Meijer grocery store. Gary found employment driving a truck for a local dairy. While Carol knew that returning to Michigan was risky for her, she believed it was time for her to help her parents. They raised her two oldest children and steadfastly loved her during all the years.

Meijer required her fingerprints as part of the application process. She secretly feared this could lead the authorities to her, but did not share these worries even with Gary. As Carol and I talked about our experiences, we found some similarities in the way we handled personal issues. We both carried our burdens alone.

Carol was rearrested October 29, 2008, on her way to work. She was just a few miles from her home. Michigan and other states had launched a new initiative searching for people on the lam. Carol was not the only escapee to be returned to prison in 2008.

When Carol was arrested again, Gary felt utterly powerless and sought help from everyone and anyone. He was bound and determined to free his wife. Neighbors and co-workers came forward to support them. Carol was arrested by the Wexford County Sheriff Department and transferred the next day to Scott's Correctional Facility in Plymouth by United States marshals. Gary immediately sought a lawyer and was referred to an attorney in Howell, Michigan. This attorney, he was told, had government connections that might prove useful.

Gary scraped together every penny they had. He paid the lawyer thirty thousand dollars upfront to represent Carol. Gary signed a contract upon hiring this lawyer that stated none of this money was refundable. This lawyer advised Gary that Carol's only chance of being released from prison was a commutation by the governor.

Carol and I spoke of her probabilities of being granted a commutation. While working on my own appeal I studied the process for obtaining a commutation in the Law Library. I discovered the Governor of Michigan at the time, Jennifer Granholm, commuted the sentences of only eighteen Michigan prisoners in her previous five years in office. This was not very promising. Carol did not feel disappointed for herself, only for Gary.

Carol was willing to be patient, far more than either Gary or myself. Gary wrote letters to legislators and contacted their lawyer regularly with questions about progress in their case. In my research at the Law Library, I learned Carol would need to prepare for a meeting with a single parole board member as the first step of the commutation process. That one person would make a recommendation to the whole parole board on whether or not to proceed. If the recommendation was positive, Carol would most likely meet with three members of the board who would ultimately decide whether or not to endorse a commutation to the governor's office.

She needed to prepare. Carol had to be ready with honest answers accepting responsibility and showing remorse. She could not stand before the parole board and be emotional or afraid. She had to be specific in her answers, giving details while owning her part in the crime. She could not hide behind a faulty memory. I knew the board wanted the truth even if some of it was ugly. With my help, she began to practice.

* * *

Most of my time that I lived in Unit Two, I bunked with a young woman named Missy. Missy came to prison at sixteen years of age. She was in prison for murdering her grandmother with a prescription morphine overdose. Her grandparents had raised Missy and her younger sister most of their lives; their mom and dad were addicts. The grandmother had occasional periods of extreme migraine headaches and was prescribed morphine.

Missy was a rebellious teen and her grandmother did not approve of her wild behaviors. Missy decided during one of her grandmother's migraine episodes to sedate her more than usual. Missy and her grandfather typically took meals and medication to her bedroom when her headaches were bad. On this occasion, Missy gave her grandmother larger doses of morphine than prescribed for a couple of days hoping to have some extra hours without supervision. From what Missy told me, I believe she unintentionally killed her grandmother.

At first, no one suspected Missy of causing her grandmother's overdose. Missy kept her secret safe for a few years. Then, in an altered state of mind, Missy unwittingly revealed the truth to an authority at a juvenile facility after being arrested. The information was reported to the police. Missy was charged with murder.

The judge sentenced sixteen-year old Missy to a minimum of forty-five years, rationalizing that those were the number of years her grandmother may have lived naturally. Missy never denied she was responsible for her grandmother's death, but she never appeared particularly remorseful either. She accepted being in prison with little emotion. She justified her grandmother's death as an error.

Under the law, until the age of seventeen, Missy was to live in a single cell. Before she turned seventeen, I was approached by Ms. Flynn, the Acting Residential Unit Supervisor or ARUS, and a unit officer. They asked me to be Missy's first bunkie. They wanted Missy safe in a cell without fear of a predator or bad influence. I was their choice. I was okay with their request and welcomed getting out of my current bunkie situation. Missy and I became cellmates.

*   *   *

Gary was caring for Carol's parents, paying the bills, working extended hours, and living a lonely life. He traveled round-trip four hundred miles once a week to visit Carol. I met this special man in the visitor room at Women's Huron Valley and recognized Gary's complete commitment and devotion to Carol. Because I was a close friend of Carol's, he immediately considered me a close friend of his as well.

For Gary, there were many personal hardships involved in Carol's arrest, but one was particularly confounding. Upon her arrest, both Carol and Gary learned that her first husband had never divorced her. She was still legally Carol Hart. Gary immediately set out to find her first husband and convince him to file for a divorce.

When Carol told me about the lack of a divorce, I thought it was incredibly funny and ironic. These two God-fearing people were living in sin. I poked fun at the situation teasing Carol and calling her a polygamist. She quickly became angry and exasperated with me. I then rubbed it in by smiling wickedly at her as though she were a shameless woman. In her frustration she asked how I could possibly laugh at such a terrible situation. Luckily, her annoyance with me never lasted long. Our friendship was special. It included full acceptance of each other along with life's absurdities.

Gary shared with me in the visiting room he'd contacted Carol's first husband and asked him to file for divorce. Gary traveled to this man's home near Flint, Michigan, picked him up, and took him to the courthouse. Gary paid for the filing fee. This again made me laugh, but only Gary laughed with me. Carol did not. She was a proud woman. Gary cared not at all what Carol's situation had been before him; he just knew he loved her.

Almost a year after returning to prison, Carol received a letter from the parole board saying they were looking into her case. She was asked to take a polygraph to prove her innocence. Carol's lawyer then contacted her and said he was setting up a deposition with an officer who stayed with her now deceased co-defendant at the hospital following the incident forty years earlier. This retired officer came forward upon learning of Carol's re-arrest on the internet. The officer told Carol's lawyer that the co-defendant, Curtis, confided in him that Carol had no previous knowledge of his intent on the night of the crime.

In May of 2009, Carol was scheduled for an initial meeting with a parole board member. We began diligently preparing her for the many difficult questions that could be asked. The process was exhausting for Carol. There was so much she had buried and now found it painful to recall. I understood if this parole board member did not find her genuine and truthful, she had no chance of ever going home.

On the day of the hearing, I prayed like I had never prayed before. It had been a long time and I hoped someone was listening. I asked God to please give Carol back her life. I said a rosary for the first time in many decades. That evening, I briefly saw Carol as we passed on the walkway during dinner. We were both an emotional mess. There was no time for her to share with me the details. We hugged and cried in each other's arms. We began to realize others were noticing, which could get us in trouble, so we parted after planning to meet later in the yard. But the prison was put on lockdown that night after a prisoner burned another in a shower by throwing hot, microwaved water on her.

I found Carol in the yard the next morning and she described the hearing step-by-step to me. It was held by teleconference. She said the parole board member asked her only a couple questions and then told her he doubted if her answers were truthful. It took thirty minutes, a short time to determine her future. She told me she remembered the two important words I had spoken of so often when rehearsing for the hearing, responsibility and remorse.

Gary was with her the entire hearing. At the end, she learned she would know if the parole board was moving forward if she was scheduled for a psychiatric evaluation.

Otherwise it was over. Carol felt exhausted and defeated. The process was overwhelming for her.

We held each other's hands for strength, promising to get through this together. We knew there were people supporting each of us on the outside, but at this time we needed each other. To our relief, Carol was soon scheduled for the psychiatric evaluation. She received official news months later in August she was being considered for a commutation. A second parole board hearing, a public hearing, was scheduled. In preparation for Carol's possible release, Gary was visited at home in early January by a parole officer. He asked Gary if he wanted his wife home and told him when Carol returned, she would be on parole for four years. He told Gary to get any guns out of the house and then showed Gary an extensive report that had been compiled on him as well.

Suddenly Carol's release seemed promising and both Gary and Carol were elated. Our conversations quickly took a new direction. Carol began talking about my needs while I remained in prison and how we would stay in close touch. I started secretly thinking about losing her to the outside world.

The public hearing was held as scheduled on January 20th. Her hearing began at noon and lasted till 3:15 p.m.

She recounted later to me what she thought to be the most difficult question asked of her. One of the parole board members asked why Carol should go home instead of other inmates who had served long prison sentences in hopes of leaving. She answered she didn't know why, and she was praying for them. About thirty people were present in the hearing room to support her, including her children, family members, friends from Manton, and the retired officer who had come forward on her behalf. There was no prosecutor, but the Genesee County prosecutor's office sent a letter opposing her release. Some family members of the victim were present and voiced strong opinions that she should remain in prison. Carol prayed the kind words of support outweighed the opposition. She now had to await the board's final decision.

The next day we met again in the yard full of hope for the commutation. That was the same day I received disappointing news involving my own appeal at the Michigan Court of Appeal's level. My appeal was denied. I kept the news to myself.

Carol became moody as the days passed and she waited for the final decision. Finally, on June 8, she was called to her Unit Supervisor's office. The governor granted her commutation. Hearing the news was surreal for Carol. She had waited almost two years to find out if freedom would ever again be in her future. She was overcome with emotion and recalled little of what was told to her except that the final paperwork prepared by the parole board would take time.

Carol's temperament fluctuated up one minute and down the next until she was released. It took a while before I fully understood why. I knew Carol was anxious about going home. When in prison it feels as though life goes on without you and it is easy to question if you will fit in again. I also believe Carol began keeping one last secret. She told me of having trouble wearing her top dentures, but not of the open sores in her mouth. She wanted nothing to delay her release and a medical problem could do just that. She figured she would see a dentist or an oral specialist when she returned home.

Carol was released on July 20th. I was not ready although we prepared to say good-bye. I met her at morning chow and walked back to her unit holding her hand. I hugged her while an officer threatened to give me a major ticket for personal contact with another prisoner. I disregarded the officer, I thought, let them do their worst. Later, I watched from a window as Carol walked one last time toward the Control Center. Tears of joy for her and sadness for me streamed down my face. Once again, I was alone.

CHAPTER TWELVE

"I ask God every day to get me out of here. I thank God every day for my sobriety. I ask for God's help in putting this experience behind me while taking what I have learned and using it for good."

— Patty Steele, Journal Entry, September 13, 2013.

Carol's absence was hard on me. She'd been a lifeline during some very dark moments. Her kindness, honesty, and listening with care were rare in any situation and especially so here in the women's prison. A month passed before I received my first letter. Rather than secretly writing me without her parole officer's knowledge, Carol informed him of our friendship and convinced him that communication between us was safe and healthy. Parolees are not supposed to have contact with other felons as a condition of their parole.

Carol's letter described time spent with family and Gary. She expressed having little time by herself or alone with her husband. Something was off, the letter lacked enthusiasm and between the lines I could hear that she was exhausted. I wondered if she was pushing herself by trying to live up to the expectations of others, trying too quickly to assimilate into the free world after two years of incarceration. I missed her. She was one of the most compassionate souls I'd ever known.

After Carol left, I began spending more time with two women who lived in my unit. Stacey was just a few years younger than I was. She was in prison for embezzlement. Carrie was in her early thirties and in prison for manufacturing methamphetamine.

Carrie was a vibrant, six-foot-two, single blond with exceptionally long legs. We quickly nicknamed her Stiltz and it stuck. She had a young son at home who was being raised by his grandmother. Her imprisonment meant absence from her son's life for six years.

Stacey's background was middle-class like my own. When she was sentenced, she left a husband and a grown son at home. Her son had recently passed the bar to become a lawyer. Neither Stacey's husband nor son accompanied her to court for sentencing. They were not present to say goodbye as she was taken into custody. Her best friend, Linda, was the only person supporting her when she faced the judge.

Stacey's husband did not visit her in prison. Instead, he filed for divorce. Stacey was heartbroken. In the months at home between her arrest and conviction, her husband had never spoken of ending their marriage. For years he'd been enjoying the fruits of her on-going embezzlement. Somehow, he never questioned where all the money for trips, college tuition, homes, and cars was coming from. Now she was caught, exposed to public ridicule and he wanted to disassociate himself from her. In my mind, that qualified him as a weasel.

When I first met Stacey, she reminded me of a school teacher. She was educated, proper, and considerate of others. She was careful to follow every rule in prison and avoided stepping out of line. Stacey feared being perceived as a disobedient inmate. She preferred not to stand out or be noticed. Ironically, Stacey worked within a school system. She was a secretarial assistant to a school principal. It was from the school athletic fund that she embezzled many tens of thousands of dollars.

As I got to know Stacey, I tried to understand her motive for stealing. In the beginning she believed she could and would repay the money. She was borrowing from the fund rather than stealing, she rationalized. To justify her behavior, she told herself that others were dipping into the athletic funds as well. Stacey had a deep desire to be accepted by others. She doubted her self-worth. Money allowed her to be generous, to be appreciated for her kindness.

There was also an element of greed. Stacey wanted a lifestyle that was beyond reach. As a family they were not particularly good about saving money. Stacey cared about appearances and wanted to live in the picture-perfect home. She wanted to entertain her friends with panache. Stacey enjoyed bestowing gifts on others, especially her loved ones. She wanted her son to finish his college education with little debt.

As she took money from the school athletic fund, she discovered that it was tougher to repay than she had envisioned. Stacey doctored the books to hide the missing funds and lived with a repressed fear that an audit would reveal the truth. She'd taken a lot of money; to live with herself she somehow created a world of denial and fantasy that no one would ever notice the missing fortune.

Though she was an embezzler, a criminal, I immediately felt comfortable with her. Her obvious kindness would not allow her to purposefully do harm to any individual. Her financial indiscretions were not connected in her mind or heart to damaging others. When Stacey relived her years of theft to me, I realized she mistakenly justified her actions. She came to believe her own implausible explanations. Stacey rationalized the institution could absorb the loss. She spoke of the school rather than the parents or children. Like me, Stacey had developed a reality that allowed her to live with herself.

As our friendship progressed and we became close, we often spoke of accountability and taking responsibility. These were difficult conversations for both of us. They forced us to examine our biggest fears, including not being forgiven and abandonment. During some of our more meaningful talks, emotions ran high. Stacey shied away from the pain that the truth exposed. Occasionally, when my candor uncovered too much truth, she lashed out at me with anger and defiance. There were times when she stopped talking to me for days. Usually, all Stacey needed was a little space to tend her wounds and process the conversation. I cared about her and understood she was hurting. I had no doubt that we would have a lasting friendship.

Her predicament was ironic, as lives often are. By her own doing, Stacey created a scenario in which she stole to satisfy personal desires and enrich the lives of her loved ones. Yet these same loved ones were exposed to public shame and chose to distance themselves from her. Sadly, much like me, she discovered that some of the people you love and count on will take the easy way out and step away when things get tough.

*   *   *

Stacey, Stiltz, and I became the three buddies. We ate our meals together and walked for hours together in the yard. In the evenings, when weather dictated, we stayed inside playing cards. Usually we could find a fourth for euchre or spades, but finding an open table in the over-crowded dayroom of Unit Two was always difficult. All units in the prison were filled beyond capacity. Rooms originally built for one held two. Closets and offices were converted into additional cells and bunked as many as eighteen prisoners.

We heard that the prison was planning to introduce a new program that involved training dogs and providing foster care. The program was to be housed on the East Side of the prison complex in the Calhoun B unit. The living conditions were better on the East Side, which housed mostly lower security level one prisoners. Officers were said to be more relaxed and less punitive, perhaps because most inmates were nearing the end of their sentences and preparing to go home.

Calhoun was a newer housing unit, more spacious than any other. The cells were larger, and the unit held fewer women. The dayroom was expansive, allowing for movement and freedom. The idea of not fighting over community tables, chairs, and microwaves sounded like a big plus. We might have a better place to play cards or just hang out in the evening rather than be confined to our cells.

We all applied for the dog program. The new program supervisor and the person responsible for selecting applicants was Ms. Flynn, our current supervisor in

Unit Two. Ms. Flynn was not an officer. Her position as unit supervisor gave her authority over officers. It was her job to select appropriate inmates that would be moved into Calhoun. She was aware that we were not problem inmates and we figured this gave us an advantage in the selection process. We were hopeful, bordering on confident.

Only a few of the inmates accepted into this program would actually handle, train, and live with the dogs that would otherwise be sheltered in the Ypsilanti pound. The program was to be called Mi-Paws, which stood for Michigan Inmates Providing Assistance Work and Service. Stacey didn't like dogs and worse, she was afraid of them. With a lot of talking we finally convinced her that we all had to try.

But in prison, optimism is quickly dashed. I soon learned that to be considered for Calhoun B, inmates had to be free of any major violations for one full year. Eleven months earlier, I was found guilty of being "Out of Place." This was a major violation usually reserved for people who managed to be found somewhere they were not supposed to be on the prison grounds. In my case, I was given a ticket for being off my bunk at Count Time. It was 4:10 p.m., and I thought the officer had already made her 4 p.m. check. I was off my bunk and getting something from my desk when she poked her head into our door window. Usually this evoked a crabby or stern rebuke, but this officer felt empowered by my mistake and wrote me up. She had the authority and she shoved it in my face for a reason I could not comprehend.

I disputed the ticket with no luck. I went before a hearing officer who thought a major ticket was somewhat unwarranted, but her position called for the strict adherence to policy. I was found guilty and given one day of confinement to my cell, a negligible consequence for a major ticket.

Unhappily I accepted the outcome knowing that now I had a major ticket on my record. It was a mark against me, hopefully not one that the parole board would some-day hold against me. And, it turned out to be the reason I was left behind when Stacey and Stiltz moved into the dog program. Ms. Flynn assured me that I would be con-sidered in a month's time and I hoped. But hoping in prison is like praying in hell.

Maybe my prayers did help. It took two months, but finally I was moved. My first bunkie in Calhoun B was crazy, loud, and frightening. She was referred to by the other inmates as Outlaw. She was a lifer with a reputa-tion for being unpredictable and unstable. While bunkies slept during the night, she blasted her television rather than using required earbuds. Officers seldom admon-ished her, unwilling to set her off. During lockdown times she jumped off her top bunk and danced wildly without music all the while waving her arms erratically and shaking her fleshy, large body like a madwoman. She boisterously sang words that made no sense. She ignored my presence as though she were alone. I never knew upon returning to my cell if I would find her in a foul, twisted mood or an excessively happy one. This woman scared me.

Bunkies never lasted long with Outlaw. Prison offi-cials were fully aware of her strange behaviors, but there was little they could do with her. They kept circulating unlucky women in and out of cells with her. I was the ill-fated woman when I moved into the dog program. I lasted one month with Outlaw before addressing the problem with Ms. Flynn. I told her I could take no more and feared for my safety. She said she had no good alternative for me. If I wanted to move to another cell without delay, it would be a six-woman cell. Nothing else was available. The idea of living in a fifteen-by-twenty foot cell, bunked head-to-toe with five other women was extremely unpleasant. Disagreements in these tight spaces were common. Nonetheless, I decided it was better than one more night with Outlaw.

For months I lived in this cell. I kept to myself seldom speaking to the others. I studied and slept, leaving the cell as soon as the unit opened or when Count Times cleared. The women in this cell developed a pecking order with two seasoned lifers asserting control. Though they basically left me alone, there were times I felt extremely uncomfortable. There was a third lifer named Lizzy. She grew up on the streets of Detroit or in the hood, as she referred to it. Lizzy had no respect for laws or rules. She understood only street justice. Lizzy carried a large chip on her shoulder toward anyone she perceived as having privilege, especially white privilege. I knew her bitterness included me. I was the enemy.

The crime that earned Lizzy a life sentence was a robbery spree in the suburbs of Detroit with a male friend. The two found their victims in convenient stores and some were killed. This was not a woman who was rational. Her views were black and white. Survival of the fittest, kill before being killed, take what you want without a care for others.

Luckily, Ms. Flynn understood my need for quiet time to study and once again moved me to a two-woman cell. My next bunkie was a woman a little older than me and in prison for a fourth drunk driving charge. Lori Ann and I bunked well together until she became sick. She was an active woman and she liked to walk. We both respected each other's space. There was never a need to lock up my personal possessions. But after only a short time together she began to have stomach issues. Whatever she ate caused her pain. Over the winter months, her belly grew large while the rest of her body got thinner. Health Care repeatedly told her to drink more water and sent her away. Only when an emergency presented itself did they begin to listen to her. She was taken to the hospital for tests. At the time she looked like she was seven months pregnant. The tests results came back positive for cancer. Immediate surgery removed an eight-pound tumor from her abdomen and chemotherapy began. Lori Ann was moved to the infirmary.

Stacey and I were given the opportunity to bunk together. In a two-woman cell for the next two years, I finally felt relaxed and content. Spending time with each other was enjoyable. Neither of us worried about our possessions being stolen. We made meals and treats together. We shared everything we had as good friends do.

Stacey had two regular visitors, her best friend, Linda, and her half-sister, Char. They devotedly came to see her every Thursday afternoon. My family often scheduled their visits to the prison on Thursdays as well, so we were able to occasionally interact in the visiting room. We made efforts to sit close to each other and Linda and Char became my friends. They sent me birthday cards and Christmas presents. They offered me support and compassion.

Stacey and I had fun together. I played jokes on her and kidded her about preparing for visits. She liked to primp before going to the visiting room. She'd put on make-up and curl her hair. I watched her as she fussed with her hair, making it puffy. I'd tease her by referring to her as Miss Texas. The last part of her ritual was putting on perfume. Linda sent magazines to Stacey and from these magazines she collected perfume samples. Before leaving for a visit she'd rub the scented piece of paper all over her body hoping to smell good. Every time I found it funny.

Stacey was easy to jokingly torment when I first lived with her. She had yet to develop her voice and was cautious. During our first few weeks of bunking together she asked me about the unit's rule on bathroom use after the 11 o'clock count. The rule was no different from any other unit. It was a little bit after 11 p.m. and Stacey was on the top bunk describing her need to use the bathroom soon. She was not sure if she should ask to leave the cell.

It seemed incredulous to me that she had been in prison for at least two years and was still this timid. So, I told her she had to wait till 11:30 p.m., knowing that was not so. At 11:30 p.m., she finally asked the guard to use the bathroom and found out they would have let her go immediately after making rounds without having to wait the extra half hour. When she returned to our cell I could not stop laughing. It took her a minute and she was laughing with me. For me, laughing with Stacey was part of the healing. For such a long time I had forgotten how to laugh. Stacey was a good sport.

Neither Stacey nor I were truly invested in the dog program. While we enjoyed living in the nicer part of the facility, we turned down opportunities to care for a dog whenever they were offered. Generally, there were ten or fewer dogs in this unit of seventy women. Each dog had three people assigned to it with one person as the main handler. Most of the women wanted dogs and were eager to care for them. It gave them an opportunity to spoil and love them like children. It gave them something to nurture.

Stacey enjoyed her free time walking in the yard or working out in the Fieldhouse. She was exercising and becoming physically fit. I chose instead to exercise my leg in the yard, study for my courses, and ultimately work in the Law Library. We could enjoy the dogs in the hallways and dayroom of the unit without having to attend dog training sessions or clean up after them.

Our living circumstances in Calhoun B were the best the prison had to offer. It was the cleanest, most roomy unit where women seldom waged war upon each other. Most inmates in the dog unit maintained a respect for others or a distance when needed. All of us knew we could be removed any time without warning. There were plenty of women waiting to move in. Officers were pleased to be assigned to this unit. There was less chaos in this unit by far, which resulted in greater respect and freedom.

During my years in Calhoun B, I worked endless hours on my appeal as it moved slowly through the court system. The paralegal classes I was taking helped me more fully understand the process and sharpened my legal writing skills. I recognized my chances were slim, but I held out hope.

Stacey was sentenced beyond her sentencing guidelines, which means longer than the maximum penalty typically given for a crime and criminal history. As in my case, the prosecutor wanted to make a public statement. In her small town, embezzlement from the school fund made a lot of news. Because Stacey had been sentenced beyond the guidelines, she had an automatic right to appeal. Ineffective assistance of counsel should have been her first argument, but her family hired the same the lawyer who originally represented her. This guaranteed this argument would not be presented to the appeals court. Her lawyer was not going to admit his own lack of competency. His meager attempts to appeal the case were unsuccessful.

As our friendship grew, I took on the task of writing a Motion for Relief from Judgement for Stacey. It was her last chance to get the court to review her sentence. Like an appeal, this motion involved in-depth legal arguments backed by statutory and case law. We both knew this motion, if written by an attorney, would have greater weight in the courts. Though I worked for months on the motion, courts were far more likely to disregard documents written by jail-house lawyers, as we were called. We asked Stacey's son for assistance. As the beneficiary of so much of her embezzlement money and a recent graduate from law school (thanks to his mother's tuition support,) it seemed logical to ask. But he chose to disregard the request. Stacey was hurt.

To this day, I believe if Stacey's original appeal was written by a competent appeal attorney and included the necessary arguments, her sentence would have been reduced. Rather than six years and eight months of incarceration, Stacey more likely would have spent a maximum of twenty-three months. This was the sentencing recommendation given to the court by the report officer; their recommendations are generally followed. Impartial justice is a myth, and behind the walls of a prison there are more stories like Stacey's than most regular citizens could ever imagine.

* * *

I missed Carol. Her kind spirit helped awaken something in me. Carol encouraged me to take a chance on myself, God, and other people again. She reminded me to look for the good in life and leave the hurtful past behind. She pointed out I was allowing fear and regrets to consume me, that I needed to release them to God. Carol spoke to me of having a special gift for helping others. She reminded me of how other inmates trusted me and came to me with their most personal problems. That I made them feel safe.

Before she was released, Carol promised to see a dentist or an oral specialist when she got home. Within months she learned she had oral cancer that metastasized. That's when she stopped writing. After seeing specialists and having surgery at the University of Michigan, she received the final diagnosis. The cancer was throughout her brain. Carol lived only six months of freedom. After she died, Gary wrote to me and told me of her last days. He described how much Carol valued our friendship and how, before she passed, Carol asked him to help me if I ever needed anything. Gary addressed me as "Ms. Patty" and told me he would always be my friend. The years with "his Carrie," he said, were the best years of his life.

* * *

Each week I attended AA meetings. The meetings gave me strength and I looked forward to the insights on recovery shared by the volunteers. They were convincing me to live in the solution rather than the problem. These women were special. They made great efforts to come into the prison. They gave me hope when they spoke of their addictions and recoveries.

THE GIFT OF SECOND CHANCES

On Wednesday nights, I walked to the West Side of the prison for my 7 p.m. AA meeting. It was held in the same building as the Law Library. Most who attended these meetings quit after receiving a twelve-week certificate of completion. Others were removed from call outs upon requesting their one-year certificates to present to the parole board.

This system of removing inmates from attendance at the AA meetings was implemented to rotate new prisoners into the meetings. There were not enough groups to accommodate everyone desiring or required to attend. I got around this system by simply never requesting a one-year certificate of completion. By passing on the certificate, the prison system did not recognize my ongoing attendance. Instead, for the sake of the parole board, I gathered weekly signatures of attendance from the volunteers for six years. I was amazed that more AA meetings were not offered to fill the need for recovery support. It also amazed me that it was so simple to get around this obstacle and continue attending.

Unlike my earlier experiences with AA, my prison experience gave me hope. I desired the message and camaraderie. Every week I looked forward to seeing my new friends. It was important to me to maintain my connection with them.

*　*　*

A position as a clerk became available in the Law Library and I wanted it. The pay was good, about $3.50 per day, the experience would benefit me, and the opportunity to help other inmates with their legal issues I thought would be satisfying. Convincing the librarian to hire me was the next step. Assuring her I was the most qualified for the position was not too hard. She was fully aware of my studies and time spent in the Law Library. I took a test and was chosen.

For two years I worked in the Law Library. Before working there, I'd spent many hours researching and learning about criminal and civil law for my own appeal and the civil case that had been brought against me. The Law Library at Women's Huron Valley was made up of two rooms. One was filled with tables for work areas and a clerk's counter which contained reference books, prison policies, and templates for filing motions in Michigan and federal courts. Michigan's prison policy and directives were updated sometimes daily. There were books on divorce, child custody, and other legal topics relevant to prisoners behind the clerk's area. The law librarian's desk sat a few feet away. There was a copy machine that the clerks operated usually non-stop during every open hour. The second room was filled with legal books from floor to ceiling. It was the job of the clerks to retrieve for inmates the correct volumes of federal and state law for researching and writing legal arguments.

The Law Library subscribed to weekly and monthly legal publications. I found the information in these publications intriguing. They were written primarily for officers of the court rather than the public. They outlined ongoing legal cases currently in the state that could set new precedent or that had created news in local communities. Some included lists of names of attorneys being reprimanded by the Attorney Discipline Board of Michigan and their offenses. Often the offenses included prosecutorial misconduct, in other words, intended unethical practice. Articles described the common practice of unprincipled behaviors by officers of the court.

Since my involvement with the law began after my accident, my understanding of the legal system had changed drastically. Where once I believed the system worked fairly and equally for all, and with an agenda of seeking and bringing about justice, I was disabused of this overly optimistic and idealistic view. Where once I believed that the prison system had the capacity for and interest in rehabilitation, now I realized how little I had known.

In my work at the Law Library it was my job to help women in understanding the legal process and helping them research their issues. Inmates are guaranteed certain constitutional and civil rights. These include the right of freedom from cruel and unusual punishment, the right to due process, the right to freedom of speech, religion, and adequate medical care, the right to freedom from racial discrimination and the right to access the courts. Most women came to the Law Library to research and write appeals, to handle custody issues, and to file divorce motions. Others were looking for information to contest or appeal unlawful prisoner living conditions or misconduct tickets. They wanted answers to problems in and out of prison.

Every inmate asking for my help was a learning encounter for me. Most women had no clue where to begin when they entered the Law Library. Since there were no computers available most the time I worked in the library, directing fellow inmates to the appropriate Michigan or Federal law was a primary function of the clerks. I enjoyed my job. Often in their search, these women shared painful stories that were difficult for me to hear or comprehend.

Many women I met in prison were unable to acknowledge the harm they did to others. These women seemed immune to personal responsibility. I listened to the stories of inmates who had killed for greed. Some women wanted to be free of marriages, but were not willing to give up their homes and possessions. Others were addicts needing drugs and willing to do anything to get them. There were women who'd killed to protect themselves or their children from abuse and also those who'd killed their children while in altered states of drug use, not knowing what they had done until later. Sadly, I met a few who murdered their children intentionally after hearing voices. Their untreated mental illness ruined many lives, beginning with their own.

Some stories shocked me and challenged my understanding of the world. How can a mother allow a wheelchair-bound child to be physically and sexually abused by her boyfriend while she stands by taking pictures? How can a woman look away as innocent bystanders have their lives ended? How can a mother try to sell her children on the Internet, or put a baby into a microwave, or grotesquely abuse her own child? Sometimes I was confronted with the reality of evil and wondered how it influences the fabric of our own lives. Some women shared with me details of their crimes that left me without compassion or empathy, but I recognized they still deserved all the protections the law allowed.

My work in the library, my time in prison, also exposed me to women who'd suffered at the hands of family or partners, yet still somehow maintained a compassionate heart. One woman was sexually abused throughout her childhood. Karen's stepfather tied her up in a barn before beating her or having sex with her. Her mother knew what was happening but was not willing to rescue her. Her stepfather threatened to hurt her more if she told. He killed baby animals in front of her to demonstrate what could happen to her. Karen survived her childhood to become a drug addict, trading one set of demons for another. She lived on the streets any way she could. She stole and became a prostitute. When I met Karen, she seemed to expect little from life or people, yet she always exhibited kindheartedness. In her upbringing she'd experienced an absence of kindness and I wondered how a woman of her inner strength might have lived if someone had loved her and given her even one safe relationship.

In her words and actions, Karen often cared about others, but she didn't believe others cared about her. Listening to her story I wondered if she would ever trust another person or trust that there was goodness in the world. By comparison, I understood how my imperfect life had given me so many more opportunities for love and safety. There was so much I had to be grateful for.

Two of the women who worked as clerks in the Law Library were unusually bright, but lacking any viable supervision, took on controlling roles within the library. When I first took the position my relationship with them was amenable, but as time went on it became troublesome. These women were both lifers. One was a school teacher who had lived in the same middle-class community as my father until she murdered her husband. Though she denied she planned his death, there was much evidence to the contrary. The other owned a health care business in Florida. She convinced one of her employees to kill her boyfriend's wife who lived in Michigan.

These were complicated women who I found to have freakish control issues and intense mood swings. They were deceitful and manipulative. It took only a short time before I realized they both viewed the Law Library as their personal domain. At times they were ugly with me for not condoning their behaviors. Like children, they sometimes refused to acknowledge my presence in the room.

These women used the resources of the Law Library for their own purposes. One spent much of her time preparing her own appeal during her work day. She hoarded typewriter ribbons and other supplies meant for the Law Library patrons. One minute she was pleasant and the next she snapped at others. She quickly became irritated if interrupted when working on her own legal issues. The other full-time law clerk ran a business out of the Law Library. She wrote appeals and grievances for inmates at a cost. She ran copies for clients and undercharged their accounts, while accepting commissary items for herself in return. These women said one thing to my face and another behind my back. I found I needed to be very careful when working with them.

*　　*　　*

The dog program ran for just over two years at the Huron Valley Women's Correctional Facility with many glitches. The dogs were mostly Pitbull mixes, strong and difficult to control. Many of these animals had problems with socializing and aggression. The women had trouble handling them. The dog trainers who volunteered to come into the prison and help us learn techniques for training and dog care found it difficult to gain entry into the prison. At times they waited interminably through counts and lock-downs before finally gaining admittance only to find that the women in the program were at meals or no longer available. These volunteers endured the negative energy and discourteous manners of the guards who were disdainful of their attempts to bring a moment of kindness into the prison.

In short, the program was a bust. Few women understood how to effectively work with the dogs. Many preferred to baby them rather than train them. There were too few opportunities to exercise the animals and many of the dogs remained unadoptable. After authorities decided to end the program, they made an executive decision to turn Calhoun B into a unit for young inmates ranging in age from seventeen to twenty-one. Older, reliable prisoners would also reside in the unit as mentors. This new strategy was as well-planned and implemented as the dog program.

* * *

Stacey, Stiltz and I remained in Calhoun B while the program transformed from caring for dogs to the new youth program. Upon implementation, a large cohort of troubled women from seventeen to twenty-one were moved into the unit bringing with them a chaos of juvenile criminality. Theft in the unit became rampant. Girls began sneaking in and out of cells to steal and have sex. The officers were not prepared to police these actions and many of these inmates appeared indifferent to consequences or punishment. The unit which had once been the most coveted in the prison was quickly tainted by youthful entitlement and disrespect.

These girls, as I viewed them, were immature, disrespectful, delinquents. They thought of only themselves and the moment. The unit changed. Trash was left in the common areas, on the tables and floors. Microwaves were left dirty. Once the bathrooms had been nicely cared for; now I expected to find hair in the drains, pieces of discarded soap on the floor, and used sanitary products in the showers. Our calm dog unit was now dominated by unregulated young women who showed no empathy for each other or for those wanting to help them. The sound of angry inmates and officers yelling at each other became the norm. Each day these young women were sent from the unit into segregation for breaking major rules, only to return a few days later unfazed by the consequences of their behaviors.

Stacey, Stiltz and I were offered the opportunity to remain in Calhoun B as mentors. We were not looking forward to being in some other unit on grounds. The Calhoun B dog program had offered a moment of respite from the worst of the rings of hell. But by failing to prepare and by bringing in way too many difficult young women into the unit all at once, the powers-to-be did not consider the work it would take to build a successful program or a working culture void of chaos and violence.

Stacey and I briefly considered the possibility of remaining in Calhoun B and taking on the job of mentorship. In our cell one night, Stacey told me she believed she would be good at teaching lessons involving finances to the youth. We had been told this program would include instructions in life skills. My first reaction was to recognize the absurdity of an embezzler teaching financial management to young street criminals. I looked up at Stacey from my bottom bunk as I fought to control my laughter. She peered back at me from her top bunk with a glare in her eyes that told me she was serious.

Stacey had an amazing knack to dismiss the obvious where her crime was involved. I could empathize, but I had come to understand we must own the offenses and wounds of our past in order to move beyond them. Fears and secrets were not addressed if we skipped this step; they grew in power and in darkness. During my drinking years, I lived an increasingly bleak existence as the secrets and shame I stuffed deep inside me reinforced a continued cycle of anguish. Failing to be honest with myself kept me from changing and locked me into a cycle of ever more lying, deceit, and misery.

As bunkies, Stacey and I developed an intimate friendship. We confessed the loneliness and shame that we had not previously been able to speak aloud. We called each other out on our attempts to circumvent truthfulness. At times, our candid conversations were agonizing. In the thousands of talks we shared, we discovered that avoidance and denial had become the automatic survival response to the lives we had lived.

Together we examined our relationships with others. Both of us found it difficult to admit that we'd been hurt or disappointed by those we cared about. At times we'd both felt abandoned by the people we loved, but fought to hide away the hurt. Was it our fault or theirs? Were we not worthy of their love? As wives, we conceded the humiliation we'd caused our husbands and painfully acknowledged that our love had not been enough for our husbands to remain loyal to us. As parents, we knew we'd been poor role models. In the safety of our cell and friendship, we admitted ownership of the confusion, the pain, and the challenges we created for our children. We acknowledged dishonesty in our adult friendships. We acknowledged the countless ways we had damaged the people we loved.

In our toughest conversations, Stacey and I considered our children, considered their shortcomings and strengths and wondered what their lives might have become if we'd been different. But we weren't. We cried thinking of our children, trying to imagine how it must feel for them to have an incarcerated mother, a mother removed from society due to personal weaknesses.

As time went along, we came to recognize that compassion and empathy were necessary in all our relationships if we were going to hope for new beginnings. We had to allow for new beginnings. Denial and fear had helped to put us here, we wondered if we could find another way. We understood we had to ask for forgiveness, knowing the answer might be no.

* * *

To me, it seemed that the Calhoun B youth program was really an attempt to corral these young inmates rather than rehabilitate them. Prison authorities began to offer instructions in hair braiding, arts and crafts, and card playing as if they were serious attempts at growth and rehabilitation. I had no interest in staying in this unit and babysitting a bunch of young women who didn't give a damn about anything.

Before long, there was a radical shift in staff. Officers who once thankfully reported to duty in this unit began asking for reassignment. I knew it was my time to leave. Stacey and Stiltz also decided it was time to move on. As low-risk, level one prisoners, we hoped we could be relocated somewhere else on the preferred East Side of the prison. About this time, Stacey and Stiltz took jobs cleaning the Control Center. These positions required special authorization from the warden and paid well but had a downside. Because they passed beyond the security gates of the Control Center, they had to endure a strip-search upon re-entering the interior of the prison. This was to ensure that no contraband was smuggled in by gate-pass workers.

For me, the idea of a daily strip-search was just too degrading. I could withstand the process of a strip-search for the sake of seeing my family and friends, but not for a prison paycheck. The officers who conducted strip-searches showed no concern for our self-respect. To most of them we were just criminals, less than human. How many times can a person be treated like dirt before she wonders if it may be true?

Like all moves in prison, there was no forewarning. One afternoon I was called to the officer's desk and told to pack up and report back. It took me less than twenty minutes to strip my bed, pull my few pictures off the bulletin board, and cram my belongings into my duffle bag. Because of required pack-ups practiced regularly throughout the prison, we lived half-packed at all times.

I wept softly as I prepared for the move. Stacey was at work and I was alone in the cell. She would come back to find me gone and replaced by another. We would find opportunities to meet in the yard, but this move was the beginning of a profound change for both of us. For me, it meant I no longer had the security of a friend beside me while living in this nightmare. My friend would not be there to walk to chow with every day, to say good morning and good night.

I found a cart in the unit to carry my footlocker, duffle

bag, books, walker, television and typewriter. These were all my belongings. I could already sense myself missing the feeling of contentment knowing Stacey was on her bunk above me. The feeling of poking fun at her for continuously re-reading the *Fifty Shades of Grey* books I gave her, missing my card-playing partner and our shared enjoyment when playing spades and euchre.

Making my way to the front desk, I was told to report to Filmore B. With my cane in one hand and dragging the cart behind me with the other, I did as I was ordered and dragged my life across the yard to another corner of the prison.

* * *

My new cellmate was Lisa, fresh out of Reception, Guidance, and Counseling. She was another embezzler and because of her non-violent crime and short sentence, her security classification was already given level one security status. She was a bit younger than I was, quiet and timid, new to prison and understandably afraid. I sympathized with her insecurities and did my best to enlighten her on how to survive on the inside.

In the quiet of the cell during our first weeks together, Lisa spoke about her life. When she was young, her parents divorced. Her dad was a minister and had remarried. In his new life he fathered eight children with his second wife. Lisa was raised by her mom, but that relationship lacked closeness. She was married and had a son by a previous relationship. She worried that her husband would not forgive her for leaving him. As she told her story, there was an emptiness about her that nagged at me.

Lisa described the specifics of her crime. She embezzled from her employer for a couple years before being caught. She was not proud of her actions, but she made no excuses. Her honesty and willingness to share touched me. In response, I spoke to her about my alcoholism, my personal battles, my accident, and the death of a strong family man along with my remorse.

As much as possible I found opportunities to walk with Stacey in the yard and most of the time Lisa joined us. As a prison newcomer, she wanted to share in our strategies for surviving the contempt of the guards, the aggression of other women, the relentless rules, the sanctions, the bells, the boredom, and the unending shroud of negativity that surrounded us.

We told her to avoid appearing afraid and taught her to walk with her head up rather than looking at the ground. Avoiding eye contact with others was a sure sign of a new or timid prisoner. The perception of fear brought out the predators and there were many.

On our walks, Lisa told us about her husband, her son, and her parents. She'd been married for two years before being arrested, though she and her husband had lived together for nine years before they were married. Her husband had trouble maintaining jobs due to a criminal record from before they'd met. Lisa was the primary breadwinner. He had needed her. She insecurely wondered if that was why he had chosen to be with her. Now, that she was no longer the provider, she wondered if he would step up and find a way to stay employed. It was complicated. If he could take care of himself, would he still need her?

* * *

About a month after becoming cell mates, Lisa told me of the death of her son at the age of fifteen. His death created a void she didn't know how to fill, along with a pile of medical and funeral expenses to pay. It was after his death that Lisa began to steal from her employer. She was afraid, confused, and broke. She was so empty inside that nothing could satiate the emptiness.

As she told me about his death, she looked at me intensely and said I had changed the way she viewed his death. She had hated the person who had taken his life. The person who killed her son was a drunk driver.

I sobbed as this kind, but damaged woman explained why she had changed her understanding of his horrible death. She believed me when I said I had no intention of taking a life or hurting the many people in my life that were affected by my alcoholism. She said she felt my anguish and sorrow when I spoke of my shame and guilt. Lisa told me I deserved a second chance to find a life that included happiness.

After a lot of tears, I listened to the details of her son's death. He was outside their home, standing by the road when a neighbor known for his drunkenness ran him down with his truck. I would have understood if she hated me with a passion that did not allow for mercy. Lisa's benevolence was a gift. I couldn't fully understand it, but I gratefully, without ease, accepted it.

Despite my personal circumstances, I was coming to realize I had many reasons to feel gratitude. I had a few really good people in my life who loved me. Even in the company of inmates, I found unexpected friends. There were women in recovery who came each week to support me in spite of the demeaning process of coming into prison. They came to hold a candle to the darkness around me. Something new was awakening in me, a hopefulness that I had not known for so long and though it felt foreign, I was ready to embrace it.

My spirit was changing. And then there was another gift when Sara called to tell me that I was to become a grandmother!

CHAPTER THIRTEEN

"My new goal is to be the best grandmother I can be. To bring joy into my granddaughter's life like my grandmother did for me."

—Patty Steele, Journal Entry, August 8, 2012.

Filmore B was over the top with chaos and disorder. The unit was filled with too many women living in close quarters. There were not enough showers, phones, or common-room space. The afternoon officer, Officer Mint, set the tone in this unit. She showed up for her day, committed to doing the least amount of work possible. Officer Mint began her daily routine by turning on her radio, intending to peacefully listen to music uninterrupted. She placed signs in the inmate bathroom directly across the hall from the officer's desk instructing us not to use the hand dryers; they disrupted her tranquility. No one challenged or approached this officer unless absolutely necessary. The repercussions of her wrath were well-known.

Officer Mint worked her shift alone. Rather than perform the duties of her job herself, she assigned inmates to do them for her. She handpicked an inmate assistant who then served as her representative and delegated chores to others. Officer Mint allowed inmates to run the unit until pandemonium erupted.

The unit lacked structure. There were unclear standards for behavior and inconsistent follow-through for misbehavior. It was a recipe for pushing the boundaries. Women abused drugs with little concern for consequences. It was common to see women strung-out, euphoric, or lethargic. Women treated each other with dangerous disregard.

Personally, I became frustrated whenever I wanted to use the phone. There was no fair system for taking turns and the unit had only three indoor phones for one hundred twenty-five women. Some women took far more than the fifteen minutes allotted. When their time ended and the phone call disconnected, they simply redialed and began another conversation. No one monitored the phones. Aggressive women went unchallenged, since reminding some women of the time limit would likely lead to a face-off.

It was almost impossible to find a chance to make calls to my family and to check on Sara's pregnancy. Rather than risk a confrontation, which I would certainly lose, I found myself making phone calls outdoors in a small attached yard outside the unit. The door to this yard was close to my cell which gave me an advantage. None of the phone hogs were interested in standing outside in the elements. In all kinds of weather, I stood outside talking to family and friends unless the phone failed to work, which was often.

Trying to stay separated from Filmore B's chaos, I chose to circumvent interaction with others. I showered before most were awake. The dayroom was small and always packed, so I avoided it. I did my best to stay unnoticed and under the radar with the guards. In one way I was

PATRICIA STEELE

lucky. I left the unit most days only to return for Count Times, chow, and lock down.

My routine in Filmore helped me feel productive while passing the time. Five days a week I woke up when the unit opened at 6:10 a.m. and hurried to the shower. The walk to the Law Library was about a half mile and I trudged there with my cane in all weather. I passed the chow hall each morning but did not stop for breakfast. At 10:30 a.m., I left the library and returned to the unit for the 11 a.m. count. After the count cleared, I went to early lunch for workers and returned to the Law Library for the afternoon shift. My workday ended at 3:30 p.m. in time to return to the unit for the 4 p.m. count.

During Count Times I studied for my courses. When the 4 p.m. count cleared, I usually cleaned the cell. At night, I went to chow with the unit and hoped there might be time to walk in the yard to get some fresh air. Many days, chow took so long that our night yard privileges were canceled. If the yard opened, I met up with Stacey and others to visit and walk. Afterward I went back to the cell and studied.

* * *

My sober time had increased; I now had close to five years of sobriety. My commitment to recovery grew in strength. The past was becoming distant. Intellectually I was learning that it was okay to ask for help, but it was still very difficult to put into practice. I was changing. Some sense, thoughtfulness, and a belief in myself had begun to return.

* * *

In prison it is so easy to worry. Time can be hard to fill and the empty spaces within me invited patterns of sadness and insecurity to fill the void. Sara described her whirlwind relationship with a man my sons despised. The boys thought he was self-seeking and self-centered. I worried that this man was using my daughter. He needed Sara's help with transportation because he had no driver's license. He needed money to pay bills, and Sara told me he had used her money for his daily necessities. He already had four children and when they were with him, she shared child care.

Sara was lonely and her mother was unable to help or advise her since she was locked away in the corner of hell from which you can see the people you love but cannot get them to see you back or hear your cries. Soon after they met, she moved in with him and within a few short months Sara was pregnant.

She tried so hard to protect me from my worries, insisting she was fine. She visited me as often as she could, so I could share in her pregnancy and watch her belly grow. We talked on the phone whenever possible. I could hear in her voice that she was tired, and it was clear that she was struggling financially and emotionally.

On the day of the baby's delivery, I called from the outdoor phone in the yard and she answered her phone. She was in labor at the hospital, alone, but she expected Brent Sr. to be there soon. Sara's father had attended Lamaze classes with her, and he was her support system. After a moment, Sara began a painful contraction. She did not complain. Like mothers have always done, she focused on the delivery and the birth of her daughter. I hung up the phone feeling empty. Mothers are supposed to support their children and help them through the tough moments. For so long I drained my children rather than uplifting them. My cinder block cell gray world, my lack of freedom and history of bad choices spilled into their lives. I was not sharing the miracle of birth with my daughter. I was not by her side to hold her hand and bring her comfort. I was not there to tell her she was a remarkable person and would be an incredible mother.

A few hours later I was able to reach Sara again. Her labor had progressed quickly. Brent Sr. arrived in time to share Savannah's birth and cut the umbilical cord. I knew he would watch over the raising of our granddaughter until I came home. I was grateful for him. Though he hadn't been a hands-on father when our children were little, he stepped up to fill the void I created by being in prison.

*　*　*

When I was young, I spent many weekends with my grandmother at her apartment, basking in her attention. We slept late in the morning, stayed up late at night, ate ice cream while watching late night television, and cuddled in her big easy chair as she stroked my hair. She let me know I was loved. She held me in her affectionate arms when I was little and shared her wisdom as I grew older. I believed I was special to her, as were all her grandchildren. When she died at the age of ninety-four, I was by her side. For five days I held her hand until she took her final breath.

Now I wanted my granddaughter, Savannah Ray, to know these same precious feelings. Savannah's birth gave me a renewed motivation to fight for a life beyond prison that included long-term sobriety. Someday, I wanted my daughter to depend on me and trust my judgement. To know she was not raising her child alone, to feel safer in the world because of my love.

Stacey and Stiltz hosted a grandmother party the night of Savannah's birth, complete with food and decorations. We ate Fat Girl cookies and peanut butter fudge. Stacey cut out baby bottles and other silly shapes and put them on a table in the dayroom where we spent the evening rejoicing. The party was corny, but very thoughtful.

Secretly I worried that I had created too much distance between my daughter and myself during my worst years of drinking leading up to my accident and imprisonment. I knew she loved me, but also believed that she feared my eventual return to her life. So many times, I had embarrassed her, frightened her, ignored her needs, and consistently chosen my addiction over the motherly behaviors that would be best for my family. How might all this affect the role I wanted to play in the life of my grandchild?

It was a month before I met Savannah. It was one of those magnificent moments in life. After driving four hours, going through the visitor entry process, enduring the pat downs and checks to see if contraband was hidden under a baby's blanket, Sara, Savannah, and now Grandpa waited for me in the visitors' room. When I held this baby in my arms, looked into her big brown eyes, and felt the gentle softness of her skin, I knew my soul was linked to hers. Sara looked at me with a mother's pride as she put Savannah in my arms for the first time. In this moment, I felt the gift of my daughter's love and understood her willingness to offer me forgiveness.

Savannah's birth fortified my connection to life and my conviction to regain happiness living sober.

For the next three years, Sara drove the eight-hour round trip to the prison as often as she could so I could cuddle my granddaughter and watch her grow. We took pictures whenever possible to chronicle my time with her. These visits were wonderful and yet heartbreaking for me. Every time they left, I longed to go with them. I wanted more than a couple hours with my granddaughter. I wanted to be a normal grandmother. I longed to change diapers and rock this child to sleep in my arms. I wanted to give her baths and feed her. I wanted to know her waking smiles in the morning and her sleepy eyes when tired. Their visits were a reminder of the divide between my world and theirs.

With my granddaughter came a shift in my thinking. I was no longer beating myself up, or counting my misdeeds, or believing that surviving prison was enough for me. I began preparing to get out and to build a life in which I could be a person my daughter and granddaughter could rely upon and possibly love. Watching Savannah grow became my calendar, the timeline toward a chance to build a new and different life.

* * *

I walked around the short quarter-mile track on the East Side of Women's Huron Valley Correctional Facility a million times during those years. I walked for the exercise and to keep my leg from stiffening up. When I first began walking multiple miles per day, I had a problem with my injured knee. One of the screws in my knee would loosen and pop out about a quarter inch causing excruciating pain. Eventually I found that I could wiggle it back in place while walking on it until it maneuvered itself back into place. At Health Care I requested an elastic knee brace, but they would not give me one. As a prisoner, I was not allowed to order a brace for myself even though they were in the prison catalogs. Finally, I got lucky. Kathy, another woman with a knee injury that had resolved itself shared one with me. I simply needed something to hold everything in place until the screw was secured by healing.

By now I knew that my knee would give me discomfort every day if I did not walk. If I walked too long my ankle and knee became sore. Weather affected my leg. Rain was easy to predict by observing my knee and ankle as they began to throb. The cold made my thigh ache. The muscles that surrounded the rod from my hip to my knee hurt until the rod was warm again. One way or the other my leg was going to give me trouble each day. There was no avoiding it, and I decided that I preferred the discomfort from physical activity rather than inactivity.

About the time of Savannah's birth, I began keeping records of my daily, weekly, and monthly miles on calendars. Stacey was amused by this, but it gave me a sense of accomplishment. There were times during those years when the weather allowed me to walk more than sixty miles in a week, a lot of walking in circles. Other weeks, when weather conditions kept me inside or the yard was closed, I was only able to achieve a total of three or four miles. At first, I kept track of these miles to motivate myself, to challenge myself. Later, I wanted to know how many times I could have walked the two hundred fifty miles home to Interlochen. By my calculations, between

January 2012 and April 2015, I walked three thousand, seven hundred fifty-six miles. I could have walked home fifteen times.

* * *

Lisa and I remained cellmates in Filmore B for nine months. Although my prison life with Lisa was predictable and safe, I put an application in to the Residential Substance Abuse Treatment program.

RSAT, which no longer exists, was a federally funded program offering therapy and education for addictive and criminal behaviors. All participants lived in the same housing unit. Everyone attended morning, afternoon and sometimes evening groups. For six months women focused on understanding their substance abuse, thinking patterns, and behaviors while opting for healthy changes.

There were several reasons for pursuing a placement in this substance abuse program. First, I believed it was the only program offered at Women's Huron Valley that effectively addressed substance abuse. It was an intense program. There were professional counselors for both group and individual therapy. I wanted to learn from experts. Though I believed I had come to terms with my alcoholism and that I understood alcohol was poisonous to my body and life, I wanted every tool possible to lessen my chance of drinking again. The Residential Substance Abuse Treatment program was designed to function as a long-term rehabilitation, a place to prepare for living with a chronic disease. It was the only program that actually offered support and planning for a life after prison.

And there was a second reason for requesting this program. Only forty women were admitted into the program every three months, though most women entered prison with substance abuse issues. I hoped an early application to the program would result in a position before appearing in front of the parole board. And I hoped that getting into this program would make it more likely for me to be released on parole at the end of my minimum sentence of seven years.

Generally, most women wanted nothing to do with this program. They knew it was strict and required daily accountability. They also knew if they were unsuccessful in completing this program, the parole board would most likely give them what is called a flop, which is an extended incarceration for at least six months. Failure to complete the treatment program was viewed by the parole board as an unwillingness to commit to change. Unsuccessful women were considered to be at high risk to become repeat offenders.

None of the rules deterred me. I preferred to live in a unit that held women to some standard of behavior. I liked orderliness and accountability. I was so tired of living in environments filled with anger and fear.

Years of attending AA helped me begin to come to grips with the patterns in my life which led to my addictive behaviors. Alcoholic Anonymous helped me identify the triggers that could put me in a tailspin and taught me how to find some healing within my relationships. Yet, I had no doubt I still had more to learn about myself and my disease. My greatest dread was returning home and reverting to old behaviors. Fear was my demon; it could lead me back to taking a drink. Only the smallest amount of alcohol would renew cravings, disappointments, despair, and ultimately hopelessness. I was praying I would somehow avoid repeating the past.

*   *   *

During my years in prison, I came to accept and understand that I had a disease. To address my addiction successfully, I personally needed more knowledge of the science behind the disease along with the skills and tools to manage it. I needed the help of others. I knew I had been the person who wanted to fix herself, by herself, and had let pride get in the way. I had to become humble enough to request assistance and graciously receive it.

Willpower was not enough. I needed the support of others who understood my fears. And more, I had to learn how to face the shame and guilt from which I doubted I would ever find relief. I had to accept I would always live with a disease dormant within me and that in a moment of weakness that disease could easily wake up. And more than anything, I had to find a place of genuine forgiveness within myself. Years of living sober within the prison helped shed some of the impact of alcohol on my brain. The presence of amazing women who came each week to help others in AA had helped me find some models for recovery. Learning to trust again, with Sara and Bob, with Carol and Stacey, were part of my recovery. But the honesty of looking at myself, accepting the results of my actions without trying to rationalize it away or blame it on others, was still painful.

Change is a process, but I worried when I saw myself reverting to old behaviors such as isolating or wallowing in the darkness of my mind. Fear of rejection persisted in my thoughts. I wondered if I could endure more personal misery in the world without immediately looking for a bottle. I was not fully convinced I was strong enough. Though I believed I was on a journey of recovery, I could not predict what that meant. I could not trust that there was a sanctuary somewhere for me, a place where I would be safe. Prison was a nightmare but going home scared the hell out of me.

* * *

The living conditions in Filmore B were rough during my last few months in the unit. The bathrooms were being reconstructed due to the presence of black mold. This mold was found in bathrooms throughout the prison, and the authorities were slowly responding to the many complaints. For years grievances had been written by prisoners because of health concerns. Prison officials responded by painting over the mold, but it just grew back. After years of grievances, the problem was being addressed with the removal of walls in the shower areas and the construction of new ones.

With Filmore B's bathrooms out of commission, our unit shared Filmore A's bathrooms. For eight weeks our bathroom was under construction. We had to sign up to shower in Filmore A and wait in line to use a toilet or sink. Bathrooms that were designed for far fewer women than were now housed in one unit, now served two over-populated units.

The officers complained of the added burden. At times officers denied bathroom use, and inmates found themselves resorting to urinating and defecating in waste paper baskets in their cells. The prison responded by bringing in outhouses. These were placed in the small yards connected to each unit undergoing remodeling. However, problems persisted. The prison only emptied these outhouses once a week, which was not nearly enough, and the odor was strong. Halfway through the week the outhouses were over-filled with human waste. The only upside was winter's freezing temperatures reduced the smell.

That winter our cell was always cold. Lisa and I complained as did others in our hallway. After a couple of weeks of complaining and threatening to write a grievance, we were handed a thermometer and told to keep track of the temperature in our cell. We discovered the room was never above fifty-eight degrees. The suggested solution from the officers was to move to a twelve-person cell in the same unit, which really wasn't a solution. So, we endured the cold by piling on layers of clothing. We went to sleep wearing socks, sweatshirts, hats and our coats. We shivered under the one extra blanket we were issued.

While living in these cold conditions sounds awful, it wasn't much different than many other appalling circumstances presented in prison. I practiced acceptance of what I could not control. The correction system never failed to remind me I was the person responsible for my situation. I believed that society felt the same way. And beyond that, I recognized nothing was likely to change.

Partway through the winter I developed a fever and chills that would not go away. Stacey told me she thought it was stress along with the cold. This was the only time I had been truly sick in prison. Being sick added to my worries. I had learned from others the horrible results of getting sick in prison.

After repeatedly asking for an appointment with Health Care and waiting several weeks, I was examined by Dr. Pei who told me to drink lots of water and eat a healthy diet. Eating a healthy diet in prison is a joke. Meals consisted of the cheapest government surplus food the private company that provided our meals could find. We ate cheap hot dogs and sausage multiple times a week. Bird stew was a regular meal. It consisted of tiny bits of meat and lots of gravy and other unrecognizable ingredients. Once every two weeks on Sunday we were served a meal consisting of identifiable meat, usually a very small chicken leg and thigh. Few inmates missed this dinner.

Dr. Pei ran blood tests while I was in her office. Weeks later she called me back to Health Care to share the results. I knew before talking to her they were not good. I would not have been called back if they were. She said my cholesterol level was very high. She told me my liver enzymes were double what they should be, and recommended I begin alternating Ibuprofen with the Tylenol that had been prescribed for me for all these years in prison. She also suggested I see a doctor when I got home to follow up. I would have to wait at least another year before being released.

* * *

In April of 2014, I moved to the Harrison Unit. The RSAT program was housed in this unit, but I had not yet been accepted. I was told that being a resident of Harrison helped my chances for RSAT although a recommendation must come from the parole board. One small step, I hoped, toward finding a way out of my life behind prison bars, fences, and concertina wire.

The winter was long and hard. Suicides and attempts were common in prison throughout the year, but after the Christmas holidays they usually increased. Emotional stressors were amplified. The darkness of winter and the loneliness of holidays intensified depression. Each time an inmate decided to end her life, it took only minutes for the prison population to spread the word. The prison grapevine was a swift transfer of usually accurate information. Before we were ordered to lockdown, we knew who and where the suicide took place. The state police and an ambulance were summoned. We waited in our cells to see if a coroner arrived.

The prison staff discouraged investigation or dialogue following a suicide. They attempted to hide details. Too many details escaping to the world could result in legal proceedings against the state. Suicides were particularly difficult for me when the person taking her life was young or had a short sentence. Some women tried to signal their desperate state of mind to staff, but resources were limited.

The prison had policies and common practices that amplified hopelessness. Routinely, prison staff responded to desperate behaviors toward self or others with punishment. Women were placed in four-point bed restraint or strait jackets. Some were temporarily incapacitated with Tasers to quiet them. Inmates were placed in isolation where they had minimal contact with others. Meals were brought to them and they were only allowed to shower every three days. Mental illness was compounded by isolation, frustration, and fear. The mental state of inmates in distress was left unaddressed.

My own attempts at suicide helped me understand what it was like to want to end a life in prison. For my first couple years in prison, I was plagued by hopelessness. I wondered why lifers and long-term inmates held on to life. Afterlife or even nothingness would be better than a life of incarceration. At least there would be peace.

That winter I also found my time in the Law Library to be increasingly challenging. I asked Ms. Franz, the librarian and my boss, to reduce my hours to part time. We spoke privately and I told her about the dishonesty occurring on the job, the business transactions and the deceit. I related the reasons patrons complained and wrote poor evaluations for some of the clerks. I was tired of the pretense; I was ready to quit if I couldn't cut back on my shifts. I'd had enough.

Ms. Franz already knew there were problems among the clerks. She heard the rumors and read the evaluations, but had ignored them. She worried the Law Library would not run as smoothly without the two women who were the source of the greatest problems. Asking me not to leave, she promised to make changes. Ms. Franz was a gentle woman who avoided conflict. Nothing changed.

It wasn't long before one of my co-workers somehow learned of the conversation I had with Ms. Franz. One morning as I was working at the clerk's desk, I scooted back my chair to get up and accidentally bumped Jan, knocking her backward. This was a common spot of congestion along a narrow walkway. We all knew to be careful when walking through this area behind someone sitting. My angry co-worker was intent on retaliation and screamed loudly for all to hear that I had intentionally tried to hurt her. She knew this was a lie, but she was aware that her accusation was powerful. If not rejected immediately, I could go into segregation until an investigation took place including viewing the video of the library cameras. That might take days or a week.

That morning, Level Four inmates were in the Law Library. Many witnessed the incident and they saved me that day. They recognized Jan used this opportunity to falsely accuse me of an assault. The Level Four inmates immediately defended me to Ms. Franz, who did not see the incident. Ms. Franz knew that Jan's false accusation could land me in segregation, and would be a black mark on my record when I stood before the parole board. She did not call officers but instead took Jan aside and spoke privately with her. This attempt had not worked, but I was concerned that I would not be so fortunate to have witnesses speak up the next time.

* * *

Throughout the winter I worried about my home and my adult children. Sara was no longer living with Savannah's father. Before Savannah was born, Sara moved back into my house, but she tried to hang on to the relationship. For a while she was moving back and forth with the boyfriend. Finally, the relationship ended when she discovered he was cheating on her.

After that, Sara and Savannah were living in my house with Robert and his girlfriend, Amy, along with her two young children. Before I left for prison and over the years, I spoke with Robert about what I wanted for my home. Above all I wanted it to remain available to all my children. I wanted each of them to know they had a safe place if needed even though I wasn't there. Unfortunately, soon after Sara and Savannah moved in, both my grown children began complaining to me about the other.

Sara and Savannah were living in the basement. Everyone shared the first-floor living area, kitchen and bath. Robert, Amy and her kids occupied the upstairs bedrooms and bathrooms. Robert spoke to me of the burden of providing for his sister and niece. He complained to me that Sara was not helpful around the house and was not pitching in with expenses. She was disrupting his life.

Sara found fault in Robert's high-handedness, his unkind words and lack of compassion. From afar I tried to settle disputes, but it was pointless. I was disappointed that Robert and Sara could not find a way to support each other and live peacefully together.

Robert and Amy had only recently begun living together and were still solidifying their relationship. Sara was struggling financially. She worked at Subway for little pay. She was unable to afford her vehicle payments and her van was repossessed. She needed rides to get anywhere.

My daughter needed help caring for Savannah, but she wasn't good at expressing gratitude and appreciation. She feared criticism. Like me she was insecure about asking for help and saw it as a weakness. She was a single mother in a crisis of her own. She was struggling monetarily and emotionally.

I struggled with feeling Robert was ungrateful for the opportunity to live at home. The comforts were many and the costs were small in comparison to renting a place on his own. Sometimes Robert reminded me that he was the only child willing or able to take on the responsibility for my property when I went to prison. He was only nineteen when I was incarcerated. I selfishly hoped Robert was taking good care of the house out of love for me. I dreamed of returning to my home someday, a home that offered a distant memory of security and tranquility.

Brent Sr. stepped in as babysitter for Savannah when Sara worked. His voice lightened up when speaking to me about her. He watched Savannah at my house. He saw a lot of Robert, Amy and the kids. He enjoyed the connection he now had with the family.

One night in an outburst of anger, Robert told Sara to leave. She was hurt and infuriated by his belief that he had authority over her. Sara knew how strongly I wanted the house to be a safe haven for all of them. But she decided she could no longer remain there.

The helplessness I felt was overwhelming. In my cell at night I was dreaming of a new life, one in which I could build the connections I'd damaged, find some safety for myself, and build a connection with the granddaughter I loved. Somewhere in my sense of myself, I was the matriarch of the family. I solved problems, the role model, the go-to person. Until, that is, I was no longer any of those things.

At my request, Brent Sr. went to the house the next day. Rather than deal with the conflict, he asked Sara to move in with him. This offered the easiest option. I had a difficult time accepting Robert's behavior. He defied my wishes as his mother; as the homeowner I felt helpless. I had given him money for house expenses. His college tuition was supplemented with an educational trust set up by his grandfather. He'd stepped up to a lot of responsibility when I went to prison, but now he'd failed to protect my daughter and granddaughter. I wondered what it would take for everyone to forgive each other and move on.

I had a feeling that it would take a lot of work and a long time for my family to heal from the wreckage of my alcoholism.

CHAPTER FOURTEEN

"The women spoke of their pain as adults and children. I was raped, I was a heroin addict. I didn't know I was pregnant until I was seven months along. The rapist left me for dead in an alley. I have come to prison repeatedly; my children were taken from me. I hope I can be forgiven someday."
–Patty Steele, Journal Entry, September 25, 2014.

My introduction to the Harrison B unit was placement in a newly converted sixteen-person cell. Women like me who requested the Residential Substance Abuse Treatment program were placed together to await a decision regarding whether or not we were contenders for this program. First, we had to appear before the parole board which would determine our readiness for parole and consider our application to the RSAT program. We had no idea how long it would be.

Hearings were slated for six months before a first possible release date and my earliest release date was estimated to be April 2015. None of the sixteen women in this cell wanted this living environment, but all of us believed the parole board would require us to attend and succeed in the program as a precondition for parole. We expected to move into two- or three-person cells after being accepted.

Our large cell contained no desks or chairs. There was only enough room for the bunk beds, like a crowded army barracks. That meant another inmate lay on a bunk just inches above you or below you and next to you on both sides within arm's reach, unless you were lucky enough to get a bed next to a wall. There was no personal space at all. I found it impossible to relax, to let my guard down, or to pray. I felt continuously on alert, watchful of others around me and ready to act.

There were no hook-ups for televisions, no diversions available in the cell. Each person was assigned a small locker stacked at the end of their bunk. The locker was not big enough to hold our state-issued property, much less our personal items. Yet we were required to have all personal property stored neatly out of sight, including basic items such as hair brushes, soap, and state-issued toilet paper. Most of our belongings were stashed under the bunks. Every time I needed to retrieve clothing or a book, I had to rearrange my assigned locker or pull out my foot locker from under the bed and dig through the contents.

Overhead lights in this cell were turned on the moment the unit opened in the morning at 6 a.m. They never went off until 11 p.m. Movement within the cell was impossible. The moment I saw this crowded, restricted space, I wondered how I would be able to read and concentrate to finish up the college classes I was taking. I was working on the principles of business management and Constitutional law. Both classes required time and serious effort. Constitutional law was especially challenging. The class examined the origins of current law and an understanding of the evolution of federal case law and precedents. The readings were complex, and the exams were the most difficult I had faced since taking classes in prison. At the same time I had to write many papers for the business course. I could not imagine finding quiet time for studying in my new cell, much less an opportunity to type a paper without the continual tap-tap-tap on my old-fashioned electronic typewriter becoming an issue for my fifteen bunkies.

My challenge was figuring out a way to complete these classes while living in a crowded cell with no privacy and filled with a lot of noise and commotion. I'd put great effort into every class I'd taken while in prison, beginning in the spring of 2011. More than three years later, my grade point average was a 4.0 and I wanted to maintain it. I needed a quiet space to study, a place where I could focus on the completion of these classes. I needed somewhere I could get my colleges classes done.

My college success in prison played a significant role in my personal narrative that I was creating a new life plan. After getting out of prison, I planned to complete my bachelor's degree. While I wasn't sure what type of work I hoped to do in the future, I discovered a keen interest in the law. I liked educating and advocating for people who did not understand the law and its complex processes. My own lack of knowledge had served me poorly and I liked supporting people in their search for legal resolutions.

By this time, I helped prepare a number of women for parole board hearings. Carol was the first and after her release other women approached me to coach them as well. I was known among many as a person who could be trusted. Generally, I could work with someone without judgement or criticism. The process of sharing honestly with me was the first step in preparation for truthfully responding to the questions of the parole board.

When coaching women, I stressed their presentation must be sincere. Once I knew the specifics of their crime, I tutored them in questions to expect and how to present their answers in the best light. Some women found it humiliating to tell the honest truth. I explained if the parole board believed that an inmate was soul-searching in good faith and sincerely wanted to change, their hearing was much more likely to be successful. Every woman whom I helped prepare received their parole.

There were only two women I refused to help. Both were unwilling to take responsibility for their crimes, even with me. They held onto their secrets, afraid to face reality. I could sympathize; not very long ago this was me. My long talks with Carol and Stacey and sometimes with Bob helped me come to grips with personal honesty and tragedy. But it was still difficult most of the time. Both of the women I declined to help ultimately failed RSAT and were denied early parole. Thankfully, most of the women who asked for my help were more willing to be forthcoming.

One woman was a special experience for me. Moe had been incarcerated for more than nineteen years for killing a friend. She offered her alcoholic friend a place to sleep in her home after nights of drinking with no place to go. The woman would show up drunk on her doorstep and Moe put her to bed. They'd known each other for many years. Sometimes Moe gave her rides to appointments and stores after she lost her driver's license.

Many years before the incident, Moe hid a gun in her upstairs bedroom closet. The gun was legally owned and registered, but she'd never used it. No one knew of the gun or its hiding place. Moe had a disabled daughter and they lived alone in Detroit. She bought the gun for safety. Moe's daughter was in a wheelchair and unable to climb the stairs. The child's bedroom was on the first floor. Moe always believed the gun was safely tucked away from any personal danger. On the night of the incident that sent her to prison, Moe's friend woke up in the upstairs bedroom in a drunken and paranoid stupor. When Moe checked on her, she attacked. The friend grabbed a straight razor from the bathroom and backed Moe into the closet.

Moe grabbed the gun and, in the struggle, shot and killed her friend. Unsure what to do next, Moe called her brother for advice. Rather than call the police, she and her brother decided to hide the body.

In prison, there are a lot of stories which sound absurd when looking back with a different perspective. At the time, Moe could not bear the thought of being arrested and taken from her daughter.

Days after the incident, Moe shared with family members what happened. Her sister alerted the police and Moe was arrested. Her attempt to cover up the crime was the prosecutor's justification for a second-degree murder charge with a long prison term. She was given a sentence of twenty-five to forty years for second degree murder.

Listening to her story, I understood Moe had committed a crime, but I also understood her fear and her moment of panic. Moe's desire to confess to her family, while understanding that some among them would most likely report the crime, suggested to me remorse and innate honesty. She expressed no resentment toward her family. The sister who turned her in cared for her daughter until the daughter died some years later.

PATRICIA STEELE

When I met Moe in the Law Library, she had already spent long years in prison helping others as a legal writer. She prepared and researched legal documents for inmates who were deemed incapable of doing it themselves. Some of these women had learning disabilities. Others were denied access to the Law Library during their placement in segregation or quarantine. Moe was in her sixties when I met her. She was a woman of few words, but when she spoke, her deep voice captured my attention. She was direct and to the point, she made no excuses. The rare times she smiled or laughed her whole body shook. She was obviously a woman who carried a great burden for many years.

Under the rules at the time of her sentencing, Moe was eligible for parole after twenty years with good conduct. She'd never received a major ticket. During her years in prison she earned a bachelor's degree with the help of Pell grants, which became unavailable to prisoners in 1994 because of changes in federal guidelines.

When Moe came to me and asked for my help, I was honored but also apprehensive. Moe was a heavy, black woman who seldom showed emotion and I was intimidated by the responsibility she'd offered me. For weeks we met in the prison yard preparing for her hearing. Moe painfully relived every detail of the night her friend died. She went over and over it again with me until she was comfortable reliving and sharing the story. We were both blessed the day she was granted her parole. She sent me a message to meet her in the yard. Moe pulled me into her arms and drew me in a hug against her large body. She was so relieved and I felt every bit of her gratitude and happiness.

*   *   *

In the Harrison B Unit, there were mentors associated with the RSAT program. These were lifers, hand-picked to act as assistants to the counselors. They all had previously completed RSAT. There were eight of these positions, and I already knew Julie, who held one of them, from when she came into the Law Library and from the Lifer's Association meetings. Julie approached me to tell me her current bunkie would soon be leaving, graduating the program and going home. She asked me to be her next cellmate. I was ecstatic. Julie recommended that I contact the unit supervisor and she would put in her request for me to move in with her.

Julie was a young, sensible woman in her thirties. She had been convicted of murder as a teenager and was currently working on having her sentence overturned under new laws that applied to juvenile crimes. Julie also happened to be one of the major recipients of the Neal lawsuit. Bunking with her meant I would have a cell void of chaos and pettiness. I felt lucky she wanted me as her cellmate.

Mentors received extra privileges in this unit. These privileges included having a say in who they would live with. Beyond that, they were usually not subject to some of the more severe consequences handed down to establish control and impart lessons. In the Residential Treatment program, an individual's misconduct was considered everyone's problem. An individual's actions resulted in consequences for all, the theory was that peers could bring about change in each other if they all felt the wrath of the misdeed.

Peer pressure was commonly used as leverage to correct individual misconduct. Punishments such as requiring the whole unit to sit for hours in silence or bans on speaking for days within the unit were typical. If an inmate in this program was found guilty of buying commissary or personal possessions from another, full house shakedowns for receipts of personal property were typical. It was also standard to make women receiving punishments stand in front of the entire unit once a week during a morning meeting and declare their transgression. This penance continued until the counselors determined a lesson was learned by all. Fear tactics are the bread and butter of the criminal justice system, based on a premise that prisoners will behave better if they are deterred by the constant dread of authority. I had personal issues with these tactics, but my goal remained first and foremost to graduate from this program.

Mentors had influence due to their positions. They worked closely with the therapists and facilitated groups. As long as they were in the good graces of the counselors, mentors had sway with the officers and the unit supervisor as well. A mentor's request was seldom denied. I knew I had a good chance of getting out of the sixteen-woman cell with Julie's help.

After asking to meet the unit supervisor, it took only a couple days before she called me to her office. The supervisor informed me that I could not be Julie's bunkie as we both had medical accommodations guaranteeing bottom bunks for physical impairments. Julie was willing to give up her bottom bunk, but the resident supervisor would not allow it. She informed us that any change in our healthcare plan must originate from Health Care. The supervisor's solution for me was to move in with Melonie, another mentor. I didn't know Melonie, but I didn't care. I was thrilled to know I would be out of the bedlam of the sixteen-woman cell.

Word in the unit was that Melonie was a bit strange. She walked the halls with an attitude of superiority and arrogance. It was thought she was stand-offish and looked down on other women. Few people spoke to her. I did not particularly care what her personality was like. If she left me alone, I would be fine. I was ready to pack up and move.

Melonie was not much of a talker and preferred her privacy. She was in her mid-forties and incarcerated at the age of eighteen for first-degree murder. She claimed her circumstances involved an abusive boyfriend who had killed a man due to jealousy. Fear, she claimed, drove her to help her boyfriend torture this man and later burn his body. I never believed the innocence she proclaimed, however, I did sense she had come to believe it herself.

In our cell, I was happy to respect Melonie's expectation of solitude. Fortunately, nothing about my study habits, including my tap-tap typing, seemed to annoy her. Though she stayed to herself, usually perched on the top bunk, she spent many hours working on intricate and beautiful greeting cards. Cards she seldom shared with anyone.

During her many years in prison, Melonie strived for a sense of accomplishment. She had long ago taken college courses, developed her artistic talents, and now was a mentor. For me, living with Melonie was comfortable. I was not looking for a friend. And I really appreciated having a full-sized locker, a desk to work on, cable television, and a bunkie who liked a clean cell. In prison, that was good living.

My Harrison B Unit routine quickly improved after

moving in with Melonie. I got up early to beat the rush to the showers and was either on my way to work by 8 a.m. or participating in the program's morning meeting. Everyone who lived in the unit was required to be present at the 8 a.m. meeting unless they had a preapproved absence. The meeting lasted an hour and a half with many segments. One assignment included the sharing of personal favorites. This included color, tennis shoe, quote, inspirational reading, and song. It was mandatory for each person to take a turn in front of the group revealing their favorite song and singing a portion. Usually, all joined in to support the woman standing embarrassed in front of them. Another assignment was to read the day's menu for the chow hall. One particularly challenging assignment was reciting the program philosophy by memory. Being vulnerable in front of ninety peers and overcoming nerves was tough for most women. The program philosophy focused on coming out of darkness and searching for happiness. It reinforced a willingness to change by making use of opportunities presented. If someone was unable to recite the philosophy without error, they were forced to repeat the assignment day after day until they got it right. As a group, we tried to send strong positive vibes to the person with this task. Many worried about completing it. The morning meeting was designed to unify the unit, hold women accountable for their actions, and instill personal confidence.

For me, the worst part of this daily meeting was push-ups and pull-ups. Pull-ups involved calling someone out on bad behavior. Push-ups were for commending those who went above and beyond. Often women secretly became angry when being called out for bad behavior. I discovered that some women used this system to attack their adversaries. Some used the push-ups to brown-nose. When there was a serious issue between inmates that required added attention, it was addressed at a Friday morning meeting. An encounter was held in front of everyone with a counselor present. The women sat in chairs facing each other, one made a complaint and the other was forced to acknowledge it and respond. The counselor's job was to direct the confrontation and bring about a resolution along with a lesson.

Few women were prepared to be confronted or criticized publicly. Inmates who have known abuse and oppression in their lives were usually defensive. They were constantly on-guard and quick to feel under attack. This exercise was intended to teach us how to assertively confront each other without aggression. The complainant was not to be hostile. And the subject of the complaint was expected to accept the grievance and respond without anger, but with reason. Most encounters appeared resolved in front of the entire unit and the counselor. However, that was not always so. Women could be mean and calculating. They would stay silent and strike at a time when it was unexpected. Grudges held were dangerous.

After the morning meeting concluded, the women who were in RSAT broke up into small groups. Some went to Home Process with their counselor, others to groups including Seeking Safety, Anger Management, Managing Grief, Beyond Violence, Cognitive Behavior, and Relapse Prevention. These were all therapeutic groups that RSAT program participants took part in over six months. The groups were designed for learning about one's origin of addiction in order to understand pain and dysfunctional behavior and open the doors for growth and change. Because I was not yet admitted into the RSAT program,

I was free to be in my cell, in the yard if it was open, or at work.

*   *   *

I lived in the Harrison B Unit for three months before receiving notice of my pending parole hearing. My hearing was scheduled for September 11th, 2014. On that day, I would meet with one parole board member who would make a recommendation to the rest of the board. It was now time for me to begin preparing myself. It was one thing to help others get ready for their parole hearing, but another to do it myself. I was anxious, excited, and I wanted it behind me. This parole board member held my foreseeable future in his or her hands. This person would decide whether to recommend me to the RSAT program and whether I would be on schedule for parole in April.

From my experience coaching others for these meetings, I had some preparation strategies. Strong letters of support helped, especially from people who would assist in the transition period from prison to home. Bob, Polly, my new AA friends, and several others, friends and family, described in detail how they would assist and support me if I were to be released. Their letters expressed to the parole board their belief in my successful parole.

I was fretful while preparing for my hearing. This was unlike all the times I'd helped another prisoner. This was my life, my chance at a new beginning, and one I wanted so badly. And yet, I recognized underlying fears as well. Was I really changed? Would I regress into my alcoholic pattern of behavior at home in an environment where alcohol was easily accessible or would I be able to manage my disease? Did my community want any part of me?

Were my children ready for me to come home? Could I find purpose and joy in my life again?

For the parole board I assembled a file of my accomplishments. Five plus years of Alcoholics Anonymous, college credits including certifications of completing a paralegal program, a victim's advocate program, and an alternate dispute resolution program. I tried to show my time was spent constructively.

In a personal letter to the board, I expressed my sincere remorse, trying to convey the sorrow I felt for the victim and his family. I spoke of my determination to live a sober future and my desire to bring meaning back into my life. I promised to go home forever repenting the wreckage my drinking had caused.

Nothing about my alcoholism was easy for me. After all these years, it was still hard to speak the words in public that I was an alcoholic. The words sounded so final, so bleak. I feared being judged and hated for it. I was still humiliated by my actions, and I struggled. Many times, I'd admitted my shame to others in an AA meeting and in personal, intimate conversations, but they were an understanding audience. It was different with people who had not themselves traveled the dark road of addiction or did not have a connection with me. How could they understand? There was nothing pleasant for me when speaking about my active, alcoholic, destructive years. Recalling the night of the accident reopened deep wounds. I feared people thinking the worst of me.

It was complicated. I wanted to present the person I was becoming, a person with worthy dreams and aspirations despite the past. Also, I also wanted the parole board representative to clearly appreciate that I fully accepted responsibility for all the devastation I had caused.

Each petitioner for parole was allowed to bring one personal representative to the hearing, and I wanted mine to be Bob. In my view, his dignified presence, his visible sincerity, and his deep love for me would certainly resonate with the parole board member. Mrs. Mitchie, the substance abuse program director, tried to talk me out of having anyone come with me other than her. She preferred to be the sole representative for the women in the RSAT program and those hoping to be accepted. Her concern, she said, was that many of us were not objective when choosing a representative, that our choices could potentially harm us. She explained she had seen many situations in which a personal representative had marred the case of the petitioner, but I was not going to change my mind.

*   *   *

For so many years I had lived as an alcoholic often negating responsibility for the damage I was causing all around me, in my life, and in the lives of the people I loved. After a while, my life became a haze, an entanglement of unhappy events without a sense of control over any of it. I had gone far down that path of addiction.

After my accident, it was a different kind of haze. It was pain and loneliness, remorse and avoidance. It couldn't have happened that way, I wanted to believe. But it had and my fear made it worse for me. Then there was jail and prison, a different kind of denial. This can't be real. It is too awful to be real, but it was. In prison, my life became about survival and I had to face the realities of a world I could not comprehend.

Now it was different as I was facing the possibility of

release and returning to my home. I was unsure that I was ready to make safe, sound choices as a free woman. I worried my doubts and insecurities would drive me to isolation. What had I learned that strengthened me to choose differently? I'd learned to survive in prison, but I'd done nothing to ensure that I could exist outside these walls. My disease offered no guarantees that I could remain abstinent. I hated it here, but I feared who I might be out there.

* * *

On the morning of my parole hearing I dressed in my best prison-issued blues, shabby long navy-blue pants and a short-sleeved blue dress shirt worn by many before me. Still, I took particular care to be presentable. I was among a group of seven inmates reporting to the Control Center at 8:30 a.m., including four women currently in the Residential Substance Abuse Treatment program and three more waiting for a determination. We waited in the visitor room while our representatives remained patiently in the lobby of the Control Center. We were not allowed to speak with them before our hearing.

An officer sat at the desk monitoring us, so there was little talk. Like everyone, I just wanted to get the hearing behind me. The stress of the situation was building in me and I looked forward to the moment that I could hug my big brother and feel the comfort of his arms. We were told that once our hearing was over, our representatives would be cleared to come back to the visitor room for a short time.

One by one the prisoners were called into the conference room. Each interview took about half an hour.

We waited. After several women had their turn, I finally saw that Bob was sitting outside the hearing room and knew my turn was soon. Bob was dressed in khakis and a sport coat. His professionalism was apparent. We made eye contact and I thought he looked even more nervous than I felt, but the love that was in his eyes once again became my strength.

At 11:15 a.m., my name was finally called, and I joined Bob in the hallway. He gave me a quick reassuring hug and smile. We walked into the small room together, holding hands, followed by Mrs. Mitchie, the substance abuse program director. Bob held chairs for us to sit down, first Mrs. Mitchie and then me.

We sat at an oblong table placed before a blank wall screen. It was on that screen that I would remotely address the parole board representative. After introducing Bob to Mrs. Mitchie, we all sat in silence waiting for the meeting to begin. In a few minutes a woman sitting at a desk appeared before us. She introduced herself as Ms. Sampson. She was direct, but pleasant. I could see her reviewing my file before looking up and directing her attention to me.

Ms. Sampson read my charges and sentencing out loud. She told me my prison record reflected two major misconduct tickets. The first she said, was a substance abuse ticket. My heart sank. Her belief that I had received a substance abuse ticket with my charges involving alcohol could earn me an extended prison stay, a flop. The ticket she was speaking of had been dismissed. It should never have been on my permanent record. I nervously explained the circumstances. The ticket was written years earlier after an officer found Ibuprofen in my cell locker in a container other than its original packaging. I appealed the ticket and won. The resulting investigation determined that the medication was not a dangerous or controlled substance. The ticket had been dismissed. Ms. Sampson read further in the file and apologized, telling me that an error had been made. She then read the circumstances of the major ticket written for being off my bunk at Count Time. I had been rightfully found guilty of this ticket. Ms. Sampson explained to me that this ticket would have no bearing on her decision, that this offense was not a concern for her.

Then Ms. Sampson turned her attention to my original charges. After her verbal review she gave me the opportunity to discuss my history with alcoholism. I told her of the chaos and damage to others during my active disease and that I knew I could never erase the wrongs or make up for them. Nervous, but with honesty, I spoke of my remorse. With the clearest voice I could muster, I took full responsibility for my alcoholism, the accident, and the pain I had caused for the Jones family. It unnerved me to speak of the damage I'd caused. I told her I wished with all my heart that the accident had never happened, and that I was very sorry. She took me by surprise by responding with compassion. Ms. Sampson told me she understood I did not intend for the accident to occur.

In response to her question, I shared with her that I attended AA through all my years in prison and also spoke of the AA volunteer women who had written letters for me. These women became my advisors, my inspiration.

Getting into RSAT was important to me for a lot of reasons. One was that completing the program improved my odds of getting out on parole at the earliest possible date. I told Ms. Sampson how I moved into the Harrison B unit six months earlier and attended their meetings

PATRICIA STEELE

in hopes of being accepted into RSAT. I spoke of the learning opportunity for me to manage my addiction going forward. I explained I wanted every tool, skill, and strength the program could help me develop.

After questioning me, Ms. Sampson then addressed Ms. Mitchie. It was comforting to hear Ms. Mitchie offer her opinion that I was a good candidate for the RSAT program. She said that the groups and the counseling in the program would benefit me, especially in the areas of shame and guilt.

Next, Mrs. Sampson addressed my brother Bob asking him if he had anything to add. Bob described the growth and the change he had seen in me over the last six years. He told the parole board representative how I had been afraid and unwilling to speak of my alcoholism for quite some time, but how that gradually changed. He spoke of our many conversations and how I slowly opened up to him and others. Bob shared with Mrs. Sampson the college coursework I'd done while in prison to help me prepare for a different life at home. As I heard his words, tears welled up in my eyes. He described a worthy person whom he admired. He spoke of someone who deserved a second chance.

At the end of the hearing, Mrs. Sampson addressed me. She said it was obvious that I had searched my soul during the years in prison, and she recognized my efforts in preparing for returning home. There were so many challenges I would face, she reminded me, including the desire to drink. And there was the heavy weight of guilt and shame I bore because my drinking led to such a horrible accident. Speaking softly, but looking right at me from her video screen, Ms. Sampson said she believed the substance abuse program would help me deal with this

226

burden along with others. She would make a recommendation to the board for my parole as well as participation in the RSAT program. And then it was over.

The next day, Mrs. Mitchie stopped me in the halls of Harrison. Looking at me differently than before, she said that I'd done well at the hearing. She then spoke of Bob's presence at the meeting. With a smile she said that she really tried to avoid bringing relatives to the parole hearings, but this time it had worked out very well.

In September, I received my official letter of placement in the Residential Treatment program and was told to be ready to begin the program in four days. For me, this meant that in theory I could graduate from the program on April 1 and paroled thirteen days later. It was probable that my prison time would not exceed my minimum sentence. And now, there was a date. It was real and it was possible. April 14, 2015, seven months and three days to go.

* * *

It was an end of the chapter for me when I told Ms. Franz that I could work only three more days in the Law Library before beginning RSAT. It was hard for me to fully embrace the idea that my time in prison had a foreseeable end, one that was in reach. Of course, I wanted out badly, but I had no clear understanding of what my life would be like. My memories of life before prison were twofold: happy, satisfied family days and then nightmares of drunken behavior. I couldn't go back to the latter, yet doubts persisted.

I had learned another way of being and coping to survive in prison. Now there was the reality that another phase of my life was coming. It was one in which I did not understand who I was to become. I did not know how to create myself as the recovering addict and the former prisoner. It was impossible for me to not worry about what I could not predict and control.

When I learned that my counselor in the RSAT program was to be Ms. Jones, I was more than pleased. Of the four program therapists, she was the one I hoped to have as my counselor. Though Ms. Jones and I had little contact during my first months of living in Harrison B, I observed her interaction with other inmates and staff. She was a formidable woman who demanded respect. I recognized we came from different backgrounds, but I believed I could learn the most from this woman.

Tall and dignified, with long dreadlocks usually pulled back off her face, Ms. Jones represented strong principles in an ocean of indifference. In a system that tolerated evil from guards who sneered while debasing a prisoner, to the disturbed prisoners who manipulated and intimidated us all, she was different. I believed her to be in her mid-fifties, with a no-nonsense attitude, but I'd never heard her raise her voice. Always direct, but never unkind, Ms. Jones wanted us to succeed.

During my months in Harrison B, I'd noted her style and inner strength. She patiently listened, never appearing to be in a rush or uninterested. She spoke of her own recovery and understanding the pitfalls of addictive reasoning. She never blamed, but laid out the process for change. Ms. Jones believed in the potential for recovery and the joy of living it. She was authentic.

*　*　*

During the last year before my placement in RSAT, my brother and I talked occasionally of the possibilities for putting together a plan to get ready for life after prison. I generally resisted this idea because freedom still felt surreal. Until this point in my incarceration, my prison life offered little in the way of skills or counseling to learn a new way of living. My experience with AA was enormously helpful allowing me to envision a future without alcohol. My college classes were helpful. With this success I could dream of new opportunities, yet I lived within a prison system set up to punish and demean rather than teach and rehabilitate. In its present form, it operates using an Old Testament view of an eye for an eye. It's about punishment. It's about using some mystical scale of justice that hurts people to make up for the harm they have done to others. It's corrections with a stick.

To help me start thinking about release, Bob investigated professionals who might come into the prison and work with me. Believing there had to be a way to bring some help to me inside, he found a female life coach who agreed to come and meet with me. Neither of us was sure of this approach, but it seemed worth trying. I put her on my visitor's list.

On the day she came to visit, she sat in the lobby for a long time and then went through the demeaning screening process of taking off her socks, opening her mouth for inspection, and finally walking down the long hallway to the visitor's room. She waited for me. When I arrived, I noticed she sat tall without looking around or making eye contact with anyone. Obviously uncomfortable, this was not the normal setting for life coaching. It took a minute before I realized this was the woman whom I was to meet with. She reminded me of a deer in headlights, scared, in shock, sitting motionless and hoping not to be noticed by the people around her.

She was a pretty woman in her mid-thirties, dressed casually in slacks and a jacket. I walked up to her and we introduced ourselves. When I sat down, we began making small talk. I thanked her for coming. She then asked me about myself and I responded by giving her frank details that she may not have wanted to hear. I spoke of the circumstances that led to my incarceration, the hell of being there, and my worries about going home. I think she was taken off-guard by my directness and honesty.

I asked about her occupation and she began telling me how she could help me achieve my desired future through visualization and affirmations. She went so far as to tell me she had visualized her third husband. Everything from his height, his weight, his dress, and his personality. I was polite, but I found this woman's explanation of her third husband and her life theory to be ludicrous. While she appeared unable to speak of the awkwardness she felt being inside a prison, she wanted to convince me I could create a world by envisioning it, including a future mate. This idea lacked reality for me. I thought all she had to do was look around and see many people whose lives were not as they had at one time visualized.

Before the end of our visit, I knew this woman would be unable to advise me. She had no experience with addiction. She had never known anyone who had been incarcerated. My challenges were beyond her imagination or expertise.

As she was leaving, she kindly told me she would not speak of me or my situation to anyone. I instantly realized she was one of many who thought my existence and troubles should be hush-hush. I told her I appreciated her confidentiality, but it was not necessary. I explained to her my years in prison could not be a secret. Pretending my circumstances were different kept me living in denial. I had to learn to live with and beyond my past mistakes. I needed to use them to shape my future. By now, I knew honesty and responsibility were key to my recovery. If I, or anyone else, kept secrets about my life, then my shame and guilt would persist. In my mind, my future depended upon first coming to terms with my past and then finding a way to move beyond it. Secrecy indicates unrelenting shame. I did not want others or myself to carry this burden forever. The way for me to have opportunities to move beyond the past was to accept it and concentrate on moving forward. Otherwise, I would not heal and change. As she left, I thanked her for coming, knowing full well I would never see her again.

Bob was curious to hear how the meeting went and came to visit soon afterward. I told him of her apparent nervousness and her surprise when I spoke candidly about my life and concerns. We laughed together especially when I told him of her visualizing her third husband. We both understood her perspective would not meld with mine. Her skin was not thick enough to adequately give professional help to a client such as me. I needed someone who could identify with me, someone who could help perfect my coping and restoring skills rather than be concerned with the fluff of life. As I relived the visit with Bob, we spoke of how difficult it must have been for her to walk into the prison. We laughed about this eye-opening experience for her. Bob and I share a sarcastic family sense of humor. We tend to find amusement in distressing moments for others and ourselves. Our family commonly deflects pain, laughing rather than crying. We are tough rather than soft, our defense when we are uncomfortable. Bob understood there would be no further need of this life coach.

*   *   *

The Residential Substance Abuse Treatment program was the exception to the rule. It offered an intensive (prison version) addiction recovery and support process. Because completion of the program and the recommendation of the counselors mattered to the parole board, most women took it seriously. And, most of the RSAT staff was committed to helping in a way that the rest of the prison experience was not.

My peers in the program taught me by the sharing of their experiences. Their personal struggles with addiction, poverty, and desperation were both frightening and motivating for me. Their stories included the experience of abuse in every form, lives without knowing love and lives of hopeless degrading poverty. Women spoke of the pain of lost children, taken by the state or given up in hopes the children would have a better life elsewhere. Some disclosed memories of being sold for drugs, beaten and raped. Others described constant hunger and having no place to live as all their parents' money went to drugs instead of food and shelter. Many revealed the depths they'd sunk to because of their addictions, leaving their families, living on the streets, prostituting and stealing to survive.

One woman described how her father played Russian roulette with her when she was a child. He put a gun on a table and spun it. If the gun stopped spinning and pointed toward her, she was commanded to pick it up, put it to her head and pull the trigger, not knowing if the gun contained a bullet. This woman wanted to die at a very young age, but ironically it was her father who lost his life as a result of the game. The drugs these women swallowed or injected were a means to forget or numb the horror and terror of their lives.

Sitting in small groups with the women in this program helped me better understand the burden trauma brings to a person's life. They caused me to reflect more on the burdens I had given to my own children during my worst alcoholic years. My compassion and empathy for others during this process grew enormously, but I continued to share little of my own personal experiences.

In my private thoughts, I rationalized to myself that this reticence was because my problems seemed negligible compared to the experiences of these women. I had a home to return to. I had a family willing to help me establish a new beginning. Life had been kinder to me than most of my peers in the groups. I didn't want to appear arrogant or condescending. Many of these women had nothing. They would be forced to return to the same ugly world they had always known without money or a safe place to call their own. Life was so unfair. I had reasons to have hope and I wasn't sure they did. Sobriety begins with hope, I told myself.

One day Ms. Jones asked to speak with me after our Home Process group. In this group, we sometimes talked about current concerns, but we also shared very personal information about our pasts and the feelings and patterns they created in our lives.

To my surprise, Ms. Jones confronted me on my

unwillingness to open up to others. She presented me with the concept that pain was pain and mine was just as important as the pain of others in the program. She expressed that while I was well on my path to recovery, I had bypassed the first step. I wasn't sure what she meant by this. For days I thought about it. Her words, I believed, referred to the first step of the 12-Step process, which says, "We admitted we were powerless over our substance and that our lives had become unmanageable."

As I digested her comments to me, I broke the first step down into three sections, the first being "we," the second being "powerless," and the third being "unmanageable." Of the three parts, I was certain I had come to fully accept the last two. Gradually I understood Ms. Jones' point to me which was the simple "we."

I still expected to come to terms with this disease on my own. I still held to the belief that I had to develop the strength to fight off my demon alone. I had to conquer the monster. When I listened to the stories of other addicts, the benefits of seeking help from others were clear. They needed the help and support of others. They did not possess the individual strength to heal on their own.

But I remained uncomfortable and unwilling to open up about my heartache, loneliness, shame, guilt, and the fears within me. I chose to protect myself by presenting as a woman strong and recovered, without exposing the sores and scars in my heart. I did not need help. Maybe I did not deserve help. Somehow, I believed, it was my burden alone to carry and to figure out how to live with my regret and my fear.

This realization was momentous for me. If I wanted to take back the power alcohol held over me, I would have to be willing to be vulnerable and share my hidden fears. I would have to admit and speak of the doubts and fears that haunted me. I would need to trust in opening my heart and putting it in the hands of others.

Special friends and family had been telling me these past seven years that they would stay by my side; all I had to do was let them. They offered their strength out of love. But I always held back. Now it was time for me to be humble and accept love and help graciously, time to trust absolutely, but it was such a change in the inner core of my beliefs.

It was time to admit how scared I remained of this disease, of failing again, and of going home. I had lots of emotions inside that I had yet to speak of. A few I had shared with my brother. A few I had shared in AA. A few I had shared with Carol and Stacey. Trust did not come easily for me.

In the days that followed, Ms. Jones continued to challenge me to step up. I was learning that instead of using my energy for presenting false confidence, I needed to use it for addressing the personal trials that remained for me. No one could know my continued needs, my fears, or my dreams unless I found the courage to share them. I could not expect people to read my mind or understand my struggles without giving them the knowledge they existed. I had to change my thinking from "I" to "we."

In our group meetings and when she pulled me aside for more personal conversations, I could feel her heart, and wondered if I could someday be a person who could genuinely encourage others in their struggle for sobriety.

CHAPTER FIFTEEN

"I have talked a lot with others recently about going home, with family and friends on the outside as well as in here. Those on the outside see my day of release as a day of happiness and only happiness. After seven long years here, how could there be anything else? I understand that day as one of happiness combined with fear. I still see struggles ahead for me, unfathomable mountains yet to climb. Do I feel positive? Yes, but I still feel a BUT. Can I live one day at a time, let my past be what it is, and find a future ahead of me?"

– Patty Steele, Journal Entry, February 8, 2015.

My close friend and past bunkie, Stacey, began counting down the days until my release, something I was not inclined to do. We met as often as possible in the yard spending as much time together as we could. Stacey spoke happily of life beyond prison, of family, friends, future employment and rejoining society, but I was worried. There were so many things out of my control, and I struggled to trust that God and the strength of others would help me find my way.

I was especially worried about being accepted back into my community. I didn't know who would give me a job with my felony record. Applying for a driver's license was not an option until I'd completed my two years of parole, so getting around without a car would present a big obstacle. My small savings would not last for long and I wanted desperately to be independent.

Going home held so many promises and so many fears. My mind tended to focus on the negative. In my small community, would they remember me for my alcoholism and the devastation I'd caused? Would they think of me first and foremost as a drunk who caused another's death? I was afraid of not being accepted back, of being ostracized. Few of my old friends had kept in touch with me, and I dreaded running into old faces and feeling their condemnation.

How would I get to all my parole obligations? I knew Sara would help transport me, but she worked and had Savannah to care for. Brent Sr. would help, but could I ask my ex-husband to plan his days around me? After getting home, I was required to wear an alcohol monitoring device on my ankle and report every two weeks to the parole agent. It would be expected of me to take regular drug tests and attend drug and alcohol counseling. All my appointments would be located in Traverse City, a half-hour drive from my home.

I wanted to feel excitement and anticipation for my upcoming release, but the obligations and fear of failure gripped my heart and soul. Could I complete a degree to have a purposeful job that would support me? Could I restore some kind of happy, sincere relationships with my boys? Would I be good for Sara? Would Sara and I find joy in living together as adults? Would I be a good enough friend to Brent Sr. after all he had done for me? Would I find comfort in the AA community? Would I feel rejection or support from detached family members and the community? I had so many questions.

*   *   *

For so long, I had imagined sleeping in my big comfortable bed in my quiet home and hearing the rustle of the wind in the trees outside my bedroom window. I would not miss the banging of doors at 6:10 a.m., the officers yelling out demands, racing to the showers in the morning, or the tasteless food in a chow hall. Just recently I'd begun picturing a refrigerator full of delicious, healthy food and scrumptious treats available to me at any hour. Grilling dinner on my own deck with family would be a dream come true.

*   *   *

My AA volunteer friends taught me that when I could admit the whole of my past, I would find freedom to move beyond it. Acceptance, I learned, did not dismiss or negate my wrongs, but allowed me to live with them. During the long process of facing my weaknesses, the AA volunteers helped me begin to believe there were still redeeming qualities within me. This was the beginning of my healing. June, Nancy, Cindy, Dawn and the other amazing AA volunteers helped me find new determination to move beyond the past.

Trusting the process and intimately exposing myself to others was the most difficult thing I had ever done in my life. I began by writing letters to my children that expressed my deep regret and personal responsibility. I asked their forgiveness knowing I needed it and not sure if it would be given. During visits with Sara and Brent Sr., I attempted short, candid exchanges about my alcoholism and the pain it caused. These conversations were awkward and unpleasant. I knew I had to address reality, but it was still easier for everyone to ignore the sorrow and grief I had caused.

* * *

My time in the RSAT program and prison was coming to an end. I packed up my schoolbooks, legal documents, and all the cards and letters I had received over the years in cardboard boxes to mail home. I wanted to walk out of prison with as little as possible. I'd arrived at prison with only a walker and a Bible. Very little I acquired during my stay was worth taking home.

At the personal property department, I arranged for my boxes to be sent home. Afterward, when walking back to my unit, I felt a wave of exhilaration and my first real feeling that freedom was imminent. The rising energy felt like a tide going up and through me—a happiness I had not experienced in years. I had to stop and steady myself for a moment.

In her vast wisdom, my seventy-something-year-old friend from California, Polly, understood that I might feel overwhelmed and wrote me a long and insightful letter. She suggested I make a daily gratitude list and keep close my appreciation for every day and every person in my life during this transition to my future. Without uttering the word fear, she reminded me to take the time and the steps necessary to care for myself.

My children made their own preparations. Robert and Amy focused on moving into a home of their own. Sara prepared to move in with me. She arranged to take a week off work to help me settle in. She planned to drive me to the parole office, drug tests, counseling, doctor appointments and anywhere else I needed to go. Brent Jr. remained distant still, and that worried me. There remained many unspoken concerns for all of us.

None of my children addressed my alcoholism directly. They did not ask me whether I might feel a temptation to drink. My alcoholism was still an uncomfortable subject and like all uncomfortable issues, better to ignore. The family patterns continued. Although I'd spoken with each of them about my experiences with AA and some of the life lessons I'd learned, I believe that to a significant degree most people still focused on my choice to drink without fully understanding this condition as a disease.

Our patterns of communication within my family were among the greatest challenges I knew I must face. My children and I had long ago forgotten how to share personal matters with each other. Our fifteen-minute phone calls and occasional visits in prison were not enough to repair the damage I had done. Now I was returning and there was great uncertainty about the roles we would play in each other's lives. Somehow, I hoped to establish trust and then perhaps the pathway to forgiveness would be possible.

During my absence, Brent Sr. had been a friend to me like few ex-husbands. He stepped up to be an active parent to Sara and grandfather to Savannah as much as his health allowed. But now, he wanted some relief from these responsibilities. Brent Sr. tried to shield me from bad news. He did not like dealing with conflict and preferred to avoid discord. I heard in his unspoken words that he was keeping things from me.

He knew some particulars about my house that he was

aware would upset me. He knew about the ambivalence the boys were feeling regarding my return. I had once been the glue of the family, but the family structure had changed with my alcoholism and incarceration. His reluctance to be clear about his concerns added to my own.

We also had to redefine the dynamic of our friendship upon my release. I was pretty sure we both recognized that we were not meant to be a couple. There were times I suspected the kids thought we would reunite, that I would come home wanting not to be alone and their father would feel the same. However, while I knew I needed and wanted my ex-husband's friendship, I also recognized I needed to put my life, my life alone, back together. I was not willing or able to complicate the situation with a personal relationship that had once failed. I was lonely, but I did not want to revisit the past problems of our marriage.

As my release time grew closer, Bob began thinking of more immediate concerns. He contacted Robert about his plans for moving and made a trip north to check on the condition of my home. The house needed to be painted inside. He asked Brent Sr. to find a local painting crew. Brent Sr. agreed, but was not eager to take on this responsibility. He seemed to think that any needed problems could be fixed after I got home. Brent Sr. did not understand the emotional toll of this transition for me. He did not comprehend how long I'd dreamed of coming home to a place that was safe and clean, the home I remembered. With a little persuasion, he found painters and scheduled them for a week before I got home. Robert and Amy planned to be out by then.

Bob and his wife, Nancy, took care of numerous details for my homecoming. They organized and sent out invitations for what was to be a quick lunch at a nearby restaurant in Ann Arbor on the day of my release. I had hoped to meet with my AA buddies and a few new friends from the area before driving north. I wanted to thank them in person, as a free woman, outside the gates of the prison, for their special friendships. These women were happy to take time out of their day, time off work, to greet me and celebrate my release. They were willing to wait until I arrived at the restaurant not knowing what time that would be or how long I could stay. My parole instructions required that I must be at the parole officer's office in Traverse City by 4:30 p.m. on the day of my release. This meant that depending upon my actual time of release, I might only have minutes to see them before beginning the four-hour drive north.

Bob and Nancy also made a second trip to my home in Interlochen just days before my release. They spent two days repairing and cleaning my home. They bought me a new bed as a homecoming gift knowing that after sleeping on a mat for seven years the bed would be a luxury. Nancy shopped for personal items. She bought me everything from make-up to a toothbrush.

Bob had talked to me about the rapid changes in technology over the past few years. Mobile phones had advanced exponentially in my seven years in prison, as had laptops. He understood that not having needed electronic devices could present an obstacle for me. Though he knew he could not teach me all I needed to learn in a day, he and Nancy readied me with a new phone and computer. They wanted me to feel secure in the knowledge that I had everything I required to embark on this next phase of my life.

During the days before my release, I knew many of the

labors Bob and Nancy were making on my behalf. However, I did not know the many surprises that were awaiting me. Bob shared enough of his efforts with me to give me a sense of manageability and confidence that I would be okay. My big brother made it clear I was not alone. He gave me the gift of feeling secure, safe in the moment of going home. He never wavered in his bond with me during my years in prison and I was assured he wouldn't in the future. I felt protected and strong due to his love for me. I asked Bob before I got out of prison what I could possibly ever do to thank him for the devotion he had shown me. He responded he just wanted me to be his little sister and love him, he had wanted to be close for so long. I reassured him I was not going anywhere.

*   *   *

Days passed so slowly. Winter in Michigan brought the snow and cold, but I bundled myself up and walked as often as possible. Sometimes it was just Stacey and me in the yard braving the weather.

In February, Brent Sr., Sara, and Savannah planned a last visit. When I entered the visitor's room, to my surprise and joy, Robert was with them. Brent Sr. had been to an appointment with his doctor at the VA hospital in Detroit and his check-up went well. Everyone had lots to talk about.

Little Savannah had broken her arm and the cast was finally off. During the time the cast was in place, she had not been allowed to visit me. With so many two-year-old contraband smugglers, it was another prison rule for which I had little respect. Nonetheless, I hadn't seen her or Sara in months. The bone was healing well, and Sara was glad to report there were no complications.

Robert was excited to tell me about the house he and Amy were buying. He also had news about a new job he was starting. He had studied aviation in college and had accepted a job for a company based in California. He was leaving in a couple weeks for training.

We were lucky enough on this visit to sit in a corner of the room where Savannah had space enough to move around freely without bothering others. Before they left, we had one last prison family picture taken. By now I had many of them. The pictures covered my bulletin board in my cell. They recorded Savannah's life and my time with her and family, moments I cherished. They reminded me daily of what I had to gain with a sober life.

* * *

Gradually I began focusing on leaving. When I was in groups sharing details about my release, I thought a lot about how lucky I was to have a home to which I could return. So many of the other women had no such place to go when it was their turn.

Upon release, most of the women prisoners were returning to environments in which they'd felt oppressed and unsafe, without a support system in place. Some would go to live in temporary Michigan Department of Correction's housing until they got a job and saved money enough to afford rent. Many were going back without a plan to communities where criminal and substance abuse behaviors were rampant, without new work skills or personal skills. Some of the women in our group had spoken of having no one in the world they could count on. Many feared not finding an honest job that would pay their bills. Some women would leave prison with only the one-size-fits-all clothing on their backs that the prison provided, having no possessions or savings. I couldn't imagine the struggles awaiting them. They faced the world alone.

* * *

I'd been planning on giving away everything I'd accumulated over these years in prison. Although it was against the rules to share or sell possessions, I began to consider who I would pass my belongings on to. First on my list was Stacey. But she was leaving prison five months after me and there was little she needed or wanted. The only item she asked for was my watch; hers had recently broken. Stacey's fiftieth birthday was the day before I was leaving, and I wanted her to have something special from me. So, I saved my few funds and purchased some soft, Nike socks months earlier. These were a prison extravagance.

Next on my list was Gail, the woman I befriended and tutored while in Level Four. We stayed in contact over the years, occasionally walking together in the yard. Prison life was particularly hard for her. With her limited social skills and her learning disabilities, survival was lonely and difficult. I never saw her with friends, and she had little contact with family. She regularly wrote letters to her kids, but they seldom came to see her. Her family offered her no financial support. So for Gail, it was usually impossible to buy anything extra. Occasionally a Ramen noodle or a popcorn was affordable. I didn't care if she used what I gave her or sold it; I was glad to think about making her remaining two years a little more comfortable.

Gail and I made plans to meet on the walkway. There I passed her plastic bowls and a utensil called a spork for microwave cooking along with a sewing kit. Sporks were a combination spoon and fork and the only utensil allowed for prisoner use in the chow hall or in the units. Coming by a legal, heavy-duty spork that could be used for personal cooking was particularly difficult as they were no longer sold on commissary. To have one that was not bright orange and obviously stolen from the chow hall was lucky. My challenge was to pass along articles to her without being detected. A ticket could be problematic for my release. The yard was a dangerous place for many exchanges that could not be hidden on your body, since we were often searched when exiting. I was still taking a chance on the walkway.

On another day, we met in the yard. I was wearing several layers of clothing as I walked into the fenced-in area. Once there, we found a spot out of sight from the guards and cameras. I stripped and Gail put on the extra layers of clothing. This way we did not have to carry any articles in our hands nor stuff them down our pants or into arm sleeves where they could be discovered upon a pat-down. In our exchange, I passed along a pair of sweat pants and a couple of button-up state-issued dress shirts. But her favorite gift was a pink sweatshirt jacket. This sweatshirt jacket was special because it could be worn anywhere on grounds. It had snaps down the front like a coat. As a general rule, sweatshirts could only be worn in the yard and in the unit. If you were cold anywhere else, you were out of luck. But, because this sweatshirt was also a jacket, it was legal. For five years I wore it everywhere and all the time.

In our final exchange, I gave Gail a couple of long-sleeved white shirts and a contraband navy-blue head-band that could be worn under a state-issued, blue winter hat and not be noticed. These items made all the difference in the cold winter months. It felt wonderful knowing I could make her time a little more bearable. Gail thanked me numerous times. When seeing me thereafter, she always said, "Thanks, lady, thanks a lot." She called me lady the whole time I knew her. I'm sure Gail knew my name, but to her, I was "lady."

I had two more items that were particularly desirable for prisoners that I wanted to leave to the right people. I wanted them for women who had a need and could make good use of them. My black leather shoes were issued to me because of my leg injury. In my first year of incarceration, I was taken out of the prison to an orthopedic doctor and rehabilitation for my leg. The doctor prescribed orthopedic shoes and a cane for me. I was so appreciative of these thick-soled, comfortable walking shoes. They'd held up well and I took good care of them. Most prison shoes had no support and were poorly constructed. They quickly fell apart at the seams upon getting wet. Most inmates dealt with cold or wet feet throughout the year. I gave my shoes to a lifer I had known since Level Four. We often collaborated on legal work and we had lived in several units together.

A big decision was to whom to leave my personal winter coat. For only a couple of my years of incarceration, the Michigan Department of Corrections had offered warm winter jackets for sale. They were made at Women's Huron Valley and sold throughout the state prisons for about eighty dollars. For me, this meant a cost of one hundred sixty dollars because of the money I still owed for court costs. A big investment. My coat was green, well made, and as warm as any winter coat purchased from a store in the free world.

My winter coat was a wonderful investment. It had kept me dry and warm for three winters as I walked to and from the Law Library or in the yard. Prison coats were thin, offering no warmth. They soaked up the rain and dampness rather than repel it. I decided to give my coat to a fellow Law Library staff member. Diane was a legal writer and a lifer. Unlike most lifers, Diane was allowed to live on the calmer East Side of the prison. We had often walked to and from work together. It had been a long time since I had felt generous; I was enjoying it.

* * *

In the RSAT unit there was a lot of activity preparing for graduation. At the same time, I began getting call outs for prison release paperwork. The prison had to verify our transportation, and receipt of parole instructions. They had to approve our place of return and clear us medically. Social security cards were issued for those who did not have one. Each prisoner left with a new state identification card. It displayed our inmate picture and our MDOC prisoner number. This ID was a stark reminder that we were not yet free of the corrections process. We would still be in a limbo from which a state bureaucrat could yank us back for any one of a hundred violations.

Our graduation from the Residential Substance Abuse Treatment program was a moment of respectful pause. Something with value had been accomplished. It was attended by representatives of the Self-Help Addiction Rehabilitation program, otherwise known as SHAR, located in Detroit. RSAT was an extension of this organization. For many, this ceremony was a first-ever graduation. Many of these women in our group had not finished high school and this graduation held special meaning for them. I felt a sense of relief at the end of the ceremony. There were no more foreseeable obstacles to my release. I was going home in two weeks.

* * *

My final week in prison went quickly. June, one of the AA volunteers, asked me to give an open talk before leaving. Sharing my story of addiction and my hopes for the future would benefit me as well as others. A few weeks before, I had asked her to be my AA sponsor upon leaving prison, she graciously agreed. June watched many women return home only to begin drinking soon after arriving in the environment that was connected to their old patterns. Whether aiding women on the outside or accepting them back into AA in prison, June always maintained hope for recovery. We agreed to talk on the phone every morning. She had walked the path of recovery herself and understood how much this transition would challenge my recovery. For me, staying in constant contact with June was one more tool I was fortunate to have after my release.

The time arrived for the open talk. I was happy but nervous to share my story. It was my last meeting and there were thirty or so women in the group. Most of them I did not know well. For more than six years I had attended these meetings, watching women come and go, accepting their twelve-week certificate of completion or their one year attendance document and losing their pass to attend anymore. I'd never claimed these certificates knowing that twelve weeks or a hundred weeks was not enough to help me change my patterns. Maybe I was too stubborn to change more quickly, too set in my ways, or too set in my thinking. Now, I stood before them describing the pain of my alcoholism, the destruction of lives including the loss of a life I could never atone for, and for my fears and dreams for the future. Out loud, in front of my fellow prisoners, I was vulnerable.

It was hard for me to fathom as I walked back to my unit that I would not attend a meeting in prison the next week. For six years I had walked, season after season, to attend them. The path from my cell to these meetings was engraved in my bones. My AA mentors never viewed me as a failure. The story was not yet over. They understood my desire to heal and have a chance at a different life. The AA message continually reminded me that I had the power to reclaim my life with effort and support. Learning to live without drinking was the first step, then and only then, would the hard work begin.

Freedom was close and finally beginning to feel real. I would next see June and my AA friends as a free woman the day of my release. I was no longer the broken woman they first met. I had changed, I was stronger. I understood that my healing process would be a lifetime commitment and endeavor. I recognized I had to be brave and not regress once home. Returning to old behaviors such as hiding behind pain was no longer an option. I had learned that denial and defense mechanisms only prolong the agony. I had to be willing to trust the cherished people in my life, blindly have faith in them, God, and myself.

* * *

It was my last full day in prison and of course it did not go as planned. I expected to spend the morning and afternoon in the yard with Stacey. It was her birthday and I wanted to be with her. Instead, I was called to Health Care in the morning for an exit interview. A few days earlier I'd been there, but they'd failed to complete their paperwork. The call out took all morning. After lunch, I went to the yard and Stacey never showed. Stacey had become a special friend and the thought of not seeing her before I left was unsettling. We had lived together for two years during this nightmare. We shared a sisterhood, cried together, and laughed in a world that was unpredictable, frightening, and which tried so hard to suck your spirit and kill your soul. We survived together.

That night at the chow hall I finally spotted her. All day I'd been looking and asking others if they had seen her. Stacey explained she had been called out for a visit in the afternoon. Friends from her hometown had come unexpectedly for her birthday. We agreed to somehow see each other again the next morning before she went to work at the Control Center.

On my final evening in prison, Brent Sr., Savannah, and Sara were coming for a short visit. They had traveled down a day early and were staying in Ann Arbor. They wanted to be close so they could be at the prison first thing in the morning to await my release. This last visit was unlike any other. We all felt emotional, excited, and nervous. We had waited for this day to come for so long.

Sara attempted to relieve me of any anxiety I was feeling. In return, I tried to reassure her nothing could go wrong. Brent Sr. was eager to close this chapter of our lives, to leave the prison and never look back. For me, it was so much more complicated. The thought of returning to a world of color, freedom, responsibility, and choice scared me. Thinking too much about it drained me.

When they departed and after one last degrading strip-search, I returned to the quiet of my cell. I needed to be alone. The anticipation was exhausting me and turning into stress. I had expected to spend my last night in prison feeling restless, but completely blissful. Instead, I felt a heavy weight I could not explain. I didn't understand why my feelings of tension and nervousness had grown so strong and outweighed the pleasure.

For my last night of sleep, I changed into an old, tattered light blue sweatshirt and a pair of navy-blue nylon prison shorts. I then folded and placed my visiting clothes on top of my empty desk for the next morning—a pair of second-hand blue jeans bought off another prisoner, a shirt ordered from a catalog, and a newer light blue sweatshirt. My well-worn tennis shoes sat on the floor. Next to these clothes were the last few personal items I needed in order to shower and get ready in the morning. When I heard the night officer yell count, I climbed on my bunk realizing I would only hear those words two more times during the night after the thousands of times I had heard them over the years.

It was during Count Times that I usually took a few minutes to write in my journal. A few days after arriving in prison I had started keeping it and now I had three composition notebooks and hundreds of pages of lined paper filled with my scribbles. These pages were a compilation of my experiences, thoughts, and emotions of the last seven years. I had written about the prison and the people, about my disease, about friendship and trust and love. In these pages there was pain and fear, shame and guilt, and the possibility of redemption. Now I was ready to write one last entry and begin a new journey tomorrow.

I realized as I wrote my final account that my worries were always the same. Letting down my loved ones was my biggest fear. Tomorrow I would go back into a world that I no longer identified with, one now unfamiliar to me. Though I lived in a place I loathed for seven years, this had been my domain. I was afraid to go home and find the world had changed so much that I no longer belonged.

Tomorrow I was walking out of prison in recovery, but still an alcoholic. I believed I would not drink, I did not want to drink, but there was no guarantee to offer anyone, including myself. I wished I could promise everyone who had ever been affected by my disease that they would never have to fear me again, but that is not the nature of the disease. That night I lay on my bed imagining what freedom from prison would feel like, while remembering that in so many ways I would never be free. Not from my addiction. Not from the harm of my past hurtful behaviors and not from my duty to find a better way.

Like no other moment in my life, I prayed to feel connected with my family, to find a path that would let them believe in me again, to let me back into their lives as a mom, a sister, or as a friend. I prayed to be forgiven.

*   *   *

I slept little that night. In the morning I was in the

shower when I heard "Steele, report to the officer's desk" called out for the last time. As I gathered the few possessions I had left, Melonie watched me silently. We had much to say, but there were no spoken words between us. She had spoken little to me the last few days. For a brief moment I stopped considering my own fears and understood that she had watched many people leave prison expecting that would never be her fate. I couldn't imagine her sadness. Leaving the cell, I went in search of a cart to carry the box that held my journal, typewriter, and a few underclothes. With my walker and the cart, I reported to the officer's desk to get my pass to the Control Center, my gateway to the world. As usual, without any words, the officer handed it to me. As I pushed my way toward the door, I said goodbye to some of the women in the unit.

And then I waited. I'd been practicing waiting for all these years and it felt normal. The women being released that day gathered at the Quartermaster's area. Those who lacked civilian clothes would receive a pair of poorly fitted khaki pants and a tan, button-down shirt. It didn't matter if you were male or female, the prison system gave the same clothing to all. As a group, we traveled through the prison grounds one last time to the West Side Control Center. Here we would be processed out one at a time. I kept looking around for Stacey hoping to see her. Without saying goodbye to Stacey, I felt empty.

We were directed to the empty visitors' room. There was more paperwork to fill out and when completed, we sat waiting our turn to enter the visitor's screening area, known as the bubble. The limbo area between confinement and freedom. Here our belongings would be searched one more time on the astounding possibility that we might be smuggling something out of prison.

As we all sat there, a prison official approached one of the inmates. This woman was planning on returning to northern Michigan, the Alpena area. Her ride sat in the lobby. The official told her a mistake had been made, her living situation in Alpena had not been approved. The woman was young, still in her twenties. If she wasn't crying so hard, she would be pretty. She was told she would remain in southeast Michigan and reside at a Department of Corrections facility until other arrangements could be made for returning home.

As I waited, I kept an eye open for Stacey hoping even now to get a glimpse of her returning inside the prison after her work shift.

Time was dragging and I wondered when it would be my turn to enter the bubble. Just down the hallway, Sara, Savannah, Bob, Nancy, and Brent Sr. had been in the waiting room since it opened at 8:30. It was almost 10 a.m. And then I saw Stacey coming through the bubble back into the prison after cleaning the front entrance. She was waiting to be strip-searched before going back to her unit for count. We could see each other through the glass wall of the visitors' room and we both began to cry. She reached out her hand toward me with tears running down her face, I wished so badly I could run to the window or go out in the hallway and hug her and tell her I would see her again soon, that I promised to write to her even if it was against the rules. I hated leaving her behind. Right then an officer appeared and directed her to the bathroom for her strip-search. She followed and disappeared.

Several women were processed out. Finally, it was my turn to walk down the dull gray hallway to the screening room and go into this closed area with the officer. This was the space commonly used for visitor screening before entering the prison. Now it was being used for my very last inspection before exiting the prison. It was 10:30 a.m. I placed my box on a table and waited for the officer to search it. Through the glass and only yards away I could see my family standing in the lobby. They were watching me intently. I wanted to call out to them, but seven years of waiting for orders had trained me and I stood quietly, like a good prisoner, awaiting instructions.

After what seemed to be a long and thorough search of my one and only box, I was finally told I was clear to leave. As usual, there was no goodbye or encouraging words from the officer. In a separate room, another guard pushed the controls and opened the steel and glass gate which separated me from my family. The barrier opened slowly. In the lobby, my family stood gathered until finally the door was wide, and the officer indicated I could move forward.

I picked up my box and walked out of the bleakness of my past crying tears of joy. First, Sara and Savannah came to me, then the others one at a time. Everyone hugged me tightly not wanting to let go, yet in a rush to leave the shackles of the prison behind. They gathered around me as though they were protecting me and ushered me out the front door.

The first day of my new life was a beautiful spring day. A day of new beginnings. My fear diminished as we drove away from the prison; I no longer felt alone. On this day I was granted my freedom, but even more I was blessed with the love and support I had yearned for, but never known how to accept. In that moment I understood the gift of a second chance.

ABOUT THE AUTHOR

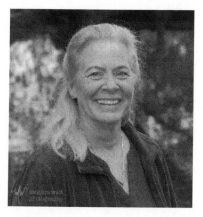

As a mother, daughter, sister, friend and grandmother, Patricia Steele understands first-hand the hardship of addiction. Patty is dedicated to helping those with addiction and their loved ones find healing and new beginnings.

Patty lives in Interlochen, Michigan, with her daughter and granddaughter. She holds a Bachelor of Science with a Minor in Addiction Studies from Western Michigan University in Kalamazoo. She is a certified paralegal and victim's advocate through Adams University in Alamosa, Colorado.

Following seven years in prison, Patty finished college and interned for three years at Addiction Treatment Services in Traverse City. She is a state-certified drug and alcohol counselor. She remains active in the recovery community by attending Alcoholics Anonymous meetings, sponsoring, and sharing her experience and hope. Patty speaks publicly of her personal involvement with active addiction along with her road to recovery. She gave a TED Talk on her experience at the 2017 Traverse City TEDx. Her talk can be seen at: The Gift of Second Chances | Patty Steele | TEDxTraverseCity - YouTube

As a mother, daughter, sister, friend and grandmother, Patricia Steele understands first-hand the hardship of addiction. Patty is dedicated to helping those with addiction and their loved ones find healing and new beginnings.

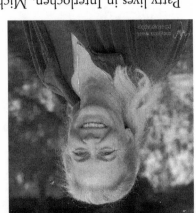

Patty lives in Interlochen, Michigan, with her daughter and granddaughter. She holds a Bachelor of Science with a Minor in Addiction Studies from Western Michigan University in Kalamazoo. She is a certified paralegal and victim's advocate through Adams University in Alamosa, Colorado.

Following seven years in prison, Patty finished college and interned for three years at Addiction Treatment Services in Traverse City. She is a state-certified drug and alcohol counselor. She remains active in the recovery community by attending Alcoholics Anonymous meetings, sponsoring, and sharing her experience and hope. Patty speaks publicly of her personal involvement with active addiction along with her road to recovery. She gave a TED Talk on her experience at the 2017 Traverse City TEDx. Her talk can be seen at: The Gift of Second Chances | Patty Steele | TEDxTraverseCity - YouTube